THE CAREGIVER'S GUIDE TO KIDNEY DISEASE

How to Support Loved Ones

James Fabin

Dadvice TV - Kidney Health Coach

Copyright © 2023 James Fabin

All rights reserved

No part of this book may be reproduced, or stored in a retrieval system, or transmitted in any form or by any means, electronic, mechanical, photocopying, recording, or otherwise, without express written permission of the publisher.

Paperback ISBN: 9798862896640

Cover design by: James Fabin

First Edition: October 2023

Limit of Liability/Disclaimer of Medical Advice

While the publisher and author have used their best efforts in writing and preparing this book, no representation or warranties exist with respect to the accuracy and completeness of this book, or that the contents apply to your current health or form of disease. The advice, research, diet, and plan may not be appropriate for all patients. A medical doctor should always assist you in making any treatment decisions, and patients should always be under the care and supervision of a physician. You should never make treatment decisions on your own without consulting a physician. Neither the author nor the publisher are liable for any medical decisions made based on the contents of this book. This includes special, incidental, consequential, or any other kinds of damages or liability.

Patients should always be under the care of a physician and defer to their physician for any and all treatment decisions. This book is not meant to replace a physician's advice, supervision, and counsel. No information in this book should be construed as medical advice. All medical decisions should be made by the patient and a qualified physician. This book is for informational purposes only.

To all the unwavering souls who stand steadfastly beside those journeying through kidney disease,

Your strength is the anchor in their stormy seas, your compassion the balm to their wounds, and your enduring presence a testament to the boundless capacities of the human heart. In the silent moments, the challenges faced, and the victories celebrated, your role remains invaluable. This book is dedicated to you — the unsung heroes who, with love, patience, and resilience, illuminate the path of hope and healing. Your sacrifices and support make the world brighter for those you stand beside.

With deepest gratitude and admiration,

James Fabin

CONTENTS

Title Page	
Copyright	
Dedication	
Introduction	1
Why Kidney Health is a Family Affair	3
My Own Journey with Kidney Disease	8
Kidneys 101	13
Overview of Chronic Kidney Disease	17
The Emotional Rollercoaster	29
Navigating Dietary Changes as a Family	35
Family Workouts for Kidney Health	47
Monitoring and Medications	56
Doctor Visits and Hospital Stays	64
Financial and Legal Aspects	77
Long-term Care and Dialysis Support	90
The Psychological Aspects of Caring for Someone with Kidney Disease	97
Employment with Kidney Disease	103
Finding Community Support	109
The Path Forward	120
Resources	127

Understanding Labs and Diagnostics	133
Important Lab Test Values	137
Glossary of Terms and Definitions	143
About The Author	153
Books By This Author	155

INTRODUCTION

Dear Reader,

Embarking on the journey of caregiving is a profound testament to the human spirit's capacity for compassion, commitment, and resilience. When a loved one is diagnosed with kidney disease, the world might seem to pivot on its axis. Questions arise, concerns emerge, and the path ahead can appear daunting. It's during these pivotal moments that a guide, a beacon of knowledge and understanding, can make all the difference.

"The Caregiver's Guide To Kidney Disease: How to Support Loved Ones" is meticulously curated to serve as that guiding light. Whether you're at the outset of this journey or further along the path, this book aims to equip you with the understanding, resources, and insights necessary to navigate the complexities of kidney disease. While this book does discuss Dialysis, it's primary focus is for caregivers of kidney patients not on Dialysis

More than just a Kidney Disease overview, this guide delves into the emotional, psychological, and practical aspects of kidney disease. It's designed with you, the caregiver, in mind. With its guidance, you'll gain not only a deeper understanding of the condition but also the tools and strategies to support your loved one in the most effective, compassionate manner possible.

This book's purpose is twofold: to enlighten and to empower. By the end, you'll have a clearer vision of kidney disease's landscape and, more importantly, your transformative role within it. Through knowledge, understanding, and empathy, together we can make the journey of kidney disease one of collective strength, unwavering support, and enduring hope.

Thank you for taking on this role, for opening your heart, and for seeking the knowledge to make a tangible difference in a loved one's life. Here's to the path ahead, to the challenges we'll conquer, and to the bonds that only grow stronger with every step we take.

Forever Grateful,

James Fabin

Dadvice TV – Kidney Health Coach

WHY KIDNEY HEALTH IS A FAMILY AFFAIR

The moment of diagnosis is a turning point, not just for the person receiving it, but for their family as well. There's an initial shockwave of emotions that ripples through everyone involved. "Kidney disease?" you may think, "What does that even mean?" The questions start racing through your mind: "How long do I have to live?", "How will my life change?", "Will I be able to work?", and "Is there a cure?".

In my personal journey, I remember feeling a profound sense of denial when I first heard the term "renal failure." Renal what? Why would it fail? The medical terminology alone can make the diagnosis even more confusing and overwhelming. Doctors, well-versed in their field, sometimes overlook the fact that these terms are not common knowledge for the average person. A diagnosis of kidney disease, delivered in medical jargon, can sound like a foreign language, exacerbating the emotional turmoil.

This language barrier can also inadvertently create a rift between healthcare providers and patients. Patients might feel hesitant to ask questions, causing important information to get lost in translation. Families, sharing in the confusion and concern, may also find it hard to know how to be supportive if they don't fully understand the diagnosis themselves.

Moreover, the emotional impact isn't solely fear or confusion; it often includes guilt, anger, and even grief. For parents, there may be guilt about any hereditary aspects of the disease.

For spouses or children, anger and frustration might manifest when the reality of life-altering changes sets in. The complexity of emotions that arise can be as confusing as the medical terminology itself.

The psychological repercussions can be equally daunting. The diagnosed individual may experience symptoms of anxiety or depression, which in turn affects their decision-making abilities and overall emotional well-being. This is a critical time when family support becomes invaluable, a topic we'll delve into later in this book.

The emotional and psychological whirlpool doesn't discriminate. It pulls in everyone—from the individual diagnosed to their immediate family, and even their extended circle of friends. This collective experience requires collective coping mechanisms, which is why understanding the emotional and psychological landscape of a kidney disease diagnosis is crucial for everyone involved.

To navigate through this initial phase, both the patient and their family need to be proactive in educating themselves. Seek out reputable sources for information, consult with healthcare providers to demystify medical terminology, and don't hesitate to ask questions—no question is too trivial when it comes to understanding your health or that of a loved one.

The Team Effort Philosophy: Everyone Plays a Role

Kidney disease is not a solitary journey. The philosophy that "everyone plays a role" is essential in managing the physical and emotional toll of this life-changing diagnosis. While the immediate focus is, understandably, on the person with kidney disease, the role of the caregiver—be it spouse, parent, child, or friend—is equally crucial.

Being there for your loved one means more than just accompanying them to doctor appointments or helping with medication. It means being emotionally present, listening, and providing a shoulder to lean on. It means educating yourself about the disease so that you can be a more effective support system. In a way, the diagnosis becomes a shared experience that requires a team effort for effective management.

Initial lifestyle changes can seem overwhelming. A new diet, medication regimen, exercise plan—it can all feel like too much, too soon. But here's the catch; these aren't just changes for the diagnosed individual. They are changes that the entire family can, and perhaps should, adopt. The recommended diet and lifestyle changes are, by all accounts, healthy changes that are beneficial for everyone involved.

You'll find that some changes are easier to make when done collectively. Take, for instance, dietary adjustments. Preparing renal-friendly meals becomes less of a chore and more of an act of love when everyone in the household is eating the same nutritious food. Similarly, exercise can be made fun and motivating when done as a family activity. This shared commitment not only helps the diagnosed individual but also fosters a healthier lifestyle for the entire family.

However, the team effort is not without its challenges. Each family member will have their own emotional response to the diagnosis and may need individual support to cope. Open communication is key. Sharing feelings and concerns can prevent emotional bottlenecks and help everyone adapt to the new normal more smoothly.

The importance of playing your part in this team cannot be overstated. Your role is pivotal in creating an environment of support, encouragement, and positivity. Whether it's adhering to a new diet, setting medication reminders, or just being there to listen, your participation makes a significant impact on your loved one's journey through kidney disease.

The Scope of the Book: What Readers Can Expect

Awareness is a powerful tool in any health journey, and this is especially true for kidney disease. This book aims to be a comprehensive guide for caregivers of those with kidney disease. According to the Centers for Disease Control and Prevention (CDC), approximately 14% of adults in the United States are estimated to have chronic kidney disease (Source: Centers for Disease Control and Prevention. (2023). Chronic Kidney Disease (CKD) National Facts. https://www.cdc.gov/kidneydisease/publications-resources/ckd-national-facts.html). With statistics like these, it's crucial to raise awareness and provide support, not just for the kidney warrior but also for their caregivers.

In the chapters that follow, we will delve into the intricacies of kidney disease management from a caregiver's perspective. We'll look at the dietary adjustments needed, the emotional rollercoasters both you and your loved one may ride, and how to navigate the healthcare system effectively. We'll explore medication management, the value of exercise, and even the financial and legal aspects that come into play.

We'll go beyond the basics. This book will introduce you to essential kidney vocabulary, help you understand lab reports, and guide you through the different types of treatments available. Consider this a toolkit equipped to help you not only understand kidney disease but also to actively participate in your loved one's health journey.

But this book isn't just informational; it's emotional too. Expect to read interviews with families who have weathered the kidney disease storm, offering insights that can only come from lived experiences. We will share resources that can offer emotional and psychological relief, and discuss how to balance work and healthcare needs.

In short, this book seeks to provide a holistic view of what it means to be a caregiver for someone with kidney disease. We'll share proven advice, personal experiences, and various resources to make your caregiver journey more informed and less daunting.

MY OWN JOURNEY WITH KIDNEY DISEASE

Life has a peculiar way of taking unexpected turns that catch you completely off guard, and this was never truer than on that ordinary day when I decided to take my kids and their grandpa out for ice cream. A momentary lapse in judgment by a reckless driver resulted in a high-impact crash into my SUV. The force of the collision not only damaged the vehicle but also inflicted lasting injuries to my back, a situation that marked the start of a long, arduous road to recovery.

For a year, I underwent therapy to correct spinal alignment issues and struggled with chronic back pain. Even lifting my small children became a Herculean task. To manage the pain, I relied on daily doses of Ibuprofen and sometimes took Advil PM to help me sleep through the night. I found relief through chiropractic care and managed to reduce my Ibuprofen intake, but the dependency never fully vanished.

A Medical Mystery Unfolds: My Body's Betrayal

One evening, almost a year after the accident, I started to feel unwell while celebrating a milestone—moving into our new home. As the night wore on, my condition rapidly deteriorated. An array of symptoms like blurred vision, persistent coughs, throbbing headaches, and uncontrollable diarrhea unleashed havoc on my body. I couldn't even hold down essential medication for blood pressure, and my health was spiraling out of control.

I visited my family doctor, but his treatments didn't help. Within a day, my condition worsened, and he urgently referred me to the emergency room. I entered the ER barely able to walk and drifted in and out of consciousness. Doctors swiftly administered potassium due to critical deficiency levels and admitted me to the Intensive Care Unit (ICU), where my new journey truly began.

The Diagnosis: Facing the Unthinkable

While in the ICU, I was visited by a medley of specialists, none of whom could provide a conclusive diagnosis. Amid my confusion and suffering, a Nephrologist finally shed light on the grim reality: I was experiencing renal failure. I remember asking what a renal was and what Nephrologist did – I was confused with these terms I was not familiar with. My Nephrologist informed me it was my kidneys. I was in denial, certain I was suffering from food poisoning. With an eGFR (Estimated Glomerular Filtration Rate) of just 8 when I entered the hospital, the Nephrologist knew it was serious and in a firm voice told me I'd be dead within 45 days without dialysis. I was overwhelmed, confused, scared, and uncertain. My wife was there by my side when I received the devastating news, leading her to go to our family doctor to check her own kidneys. I knew I had to do something so that I would be here for my family. I resolved to understand my condition better, asking questions and seeking answers. This is when I began to realize that my fight was far from over.

A Relentless Pursuit of Knowledge: My Lifeline

I refused to accept my fate passively. I spent hours poring over medical journals, academic papers, and testimonials from other patients online. I unearthed data that showcased how other countries, with far fewer resources, were achieving better outcomes in kidney care. This gave me hope, and I was determined to beat kidney disease without succumbing to the daunting prospect of dialysis.

My nephrologist was skeptical, but the research I had found offered a different path—a holistic approach, involving diet, lifestyle changes, and better blood pressure management. This beacon of hope ignited a fire within me, fueling my resolve to reclaim my life.

Taking The Road Less Traveled: Diet and Lifestyle Changes

My healthcare team and I worked closely to find the ideal combination of blood pressure medications, which helped stabilize my condition. Moreover, I implemented drastic dietary changes. These modifications were not easy, but as days turned into weeks and weeks into months, something incredible happened. My eGFR improved, and I felt stronger and more energetic. I even managed to walk up to five miles a day, demonstrating that the spirit within me was unbreakable.

During this period, I also fell prey to the allure of quick fixes and miracle cures. I questioned my doctors about every possible remedy I found online. However, the brutal reality hit me—most of these solutions were shams designed to exploit people like me. The actual road to recovery wasn't through quick fixes but through dedicated, scientifically-backed lifestyle changes.

The Role of My Family: Beyond Caregivers

My journey through kidney disease would have been incomprehensibly more difficult without the unyielding support of my family. Not merely spectators, my wife and children actively engage as integral components of my healthcare team. Often, when diagnosed with a chronic illness like kidney disease, people report feelings of isolation, but in my case, it has been markedly different.

My wife has been my rock, going above and beyond the typical duties of a caregiver. She has taken it upon herself to understand the complexities of my condition, the renal diet, and my medication. We've turned our kitchen into a dietary lab, testing recipes that meet my kidney needs but also satisfy the family's tastebuds. But her support is not just confined to the tangible aspects of care. She knows when I need emotional boosting and how to read my moods better than anyone. Her companionship has lessened the emotional burden that kidney disease often brings.

My children, young but incredibly perceptive, contribute to my ongoing struggle in ways that they might not fully comprehend. They bring boundless joy and a unique kind of emotional sustenance that only a child can offer. And let me not forget how they have become tiny but determined advocates of kidney disease awareness. They absorb the knowledge we share, internalize the importance of early detection, and become youthful heralds spreading vital information. The fact that they stand beside me helps motivate me to make healthier choices every single day.

Shared Sacrifices and Collective Triumphs

Living with kidney disease isn't just about personal sacrifices; it's often a collective endeavor that requires adjustments from everyone involved. My family has been willing to make lifestyle changes to not only accommodate my needs but also to promote a healthier way of life for everyone. For instance, we have all transitioned to eating lower sodium foods, thereby making it a family affair. These collective measures yield collective benefits. By adopting healthier habits, we not only manage my kidney disease better but also instill a culture of health and wellness in our family as a whole.

When I look back at the milestones I've achieved in managing kidney disease—every tweak in the diet, every pill accurately administered, and every dialysis session survived—I see not just my victories, but ours as a family. It's a tapestry of shared sacrifices and collective triumphs. I firmly believe that this united front contributes substantially to the improved quality of my life, offering me a treasure trove of emotional resilience and physical strength to continue my fight against kidney disease.

And so, the role of supportive relationships in managing a chronic condition like kidney disease cannot be overstated. It's a multifaceted boon—improving mental well-being, helping to stay on track with medical and dietary plans, and most importantly, nurturing the emotional fortitude needed to face the myriad challenges of living with kidney disease.

KIDNEYS 101

Kidneys are vital organs that play a pivotal role in maintaining overall health. While they often take a backseat in discussions about the human body, their importance is undeniable. In this chapter, we will explore the various functions of the kidneys and how they contribute to overall health. By understanding the role of the kidneys, you can better appreciate their significance and the need to maintain their health.

Anatomy and Location: The Kidneys' Strategic Position

The human body has two kidneys, which are bean-shaped organs, each roughly the size of a fist. They are strategically located on either side of the spine, just below the rib cage, in the lower back region. Each kidney is composed of approximately 1 million tiny filtering units called nephrons. Nephrons are the functional units of the kidneys responsible for filtering waste products, excess water, and toxins from the blood, playing a central role in maintaining a healthy internal environment.

Blood Supply and Nephrons: A Dynamic Partnership

The kidneys filter all of the blood in your body several times a day, making them one of the most highly perfused organs in the body. Blood enters each kidney through the renal artery, which branches into smaller arteries, eventually reaching the nephrons. As blood flows through the nephrons, waste products, excess water, and toxins are filtered out, while essential nutrients and electrolytes are reabsorbed into the bloodstream. The filtered waste products, water, and toxins form urine, which then flows through the renal tubules and collecting ducts into the renal pelvis. From the renal pelvis, urine is transported to the bladder via the ureters, where it is stored until it is eliminated from the body through the urethra.

The Multifaceted Functions of the Kidneys

The kidneys perform a variety of essential functions that contribute to overall health. These functions include:

Filtering Waste Products and Toxins: The primary function of the kidneys is to filter waste products and toxins from the blood, which are then excreted through the urine. This process helps maintain the balance of chemicals and fluids in the body, ensuring a healthy internal environment.

Regulating Fluid Balance: Kidneys help maintain the balance of fluids in the body by adjusting the amount of water that is reabsorbed into the bloodstream or excreted as urine. This balance is crucial for proper hydration, blood pressure control, and overall health.

Electrolyte Balance: The kidneys play a critical role in maintaining the balance of electrolytes in the body, including sodium, potassium, calcium, and phosphate. Electrolytes are essential for various body functions, including muscle contractions, nerve transmissions, and maintaining the body's acid-base balance.

Acid-Base Balance: The kidneys help maintain the body's acid-base balance by excreting excess acids or bases in the urine. This balance is critical for maintaining the proper pH of blood and other body fluids, which is essential for optimal functioning of cells, tissues, and organs.

Hormone Production: The kidneys produce several hormones that are essential for various body functions. Some of these hormones include:

- Erythropoietin (EPO): This hormone stimulates the production of red blood cells in the bone marrow,

- which helps maintain an adequate supply of oxygen-carrying cells in the bloodstream.
  - Renin: This enzyme is involved in regulating blood pressure by controlling the constriction and dilation of blood vessels.
  - Calcitriol (active vitamin D): This hormone helps regulate calcium and phosphate balance, which is essential for bone health and overall mineral balance in the body.

Blood Pressure Regulation: The kidneys play a crucial role in regulating blood pressure by managing the volume and composition of bodily fluids, as well as producing hormones that influence blood vessel constriction and dilation. In later chapters, we will explore how high blood pressure is a primary cause of kidney damage, which in turn impairs the kidney's ability to regulate blood pressure effectively. This creates a snowball effect, causing the kidneys to deteriorate progressively, ultimately leading to kidney failure.

Glucose Homeostasis: The kidneys help maintain blood glucose levels by reabsorbing filtered glucose and producing glucose through a process called gluconeogenesis. This helps ensure that the body has a constant supply of energy, particularly during periods of fasting or intense physical activity.

Metabolism of Medications: The kidneys play a significant role in the metabolism and elimination of medications from the body. They help filter out drugs and their metabolites, ensuring that the body is not exposed to potentially harmful substances for extended periods.

Urea Production: The kidneys produce urea, a waste product formed from the breakdown of proteins in the liver. Urea is then transported to the kidneys, where it is filtered and excreted in the urine.

The Critical Importance of Kidney Health

Preserving the health of our kidneys is crucial for overall well-being. Kidney disease or malfunction can give rise to an array of complications, such as:

Fluid Overload: When kidneys cannot effectively regulate fluid balance, excess fluid may accumulate within the body. This can result in swelling (edema), elevated blood pressure, and potentially fatal conditions like congestive heart failure.

Electrolyte Imbalances: Compromised kidney function can lead to imbalances in critical electrolytes, including potassium and sodium. This may cause muscle weakness, irregular heartbeats, and additional complications.

Anemia: Damaged kidneys can produce less erythropoietin, resulting in anemia. This condition is marked by a decline in red blood cell count and a diminished capacity to transport oxygen throughout the body.

Bone and Mineral Disorders: Impaired kidney function can upset the balance of calcium and phosphate, causing weakened bones, an increased likelihood of fractures, and other complications related to bone and mineral metabolism.

Cardiovascular Disease: The risk of cardiovascular disease escalates in the presence of kidney disease, owing to factors such as hypertension, fluid overload, and the accumulation of detrimental substances in the bloodstream.

Kidney Failure: Severe kidney disease can culminate in kidney failure, a life-threatening condition where the kidneys can no longer carry out their essential functions. Treatment options for kidney failure include dialysis or a kidney transplant.

OVERVIEW OF CHRONIC KIDNEY DISEASE

Chronic Kidney Disease (CKD) is a long-term health condition that impacts a significant number of individuals across the globe. It involves the slow and steady decline of kidney function, which can result in a range of health issues and eventually necessitate dialysis or a kidney transplant. In this chapter, we'll cover the basics of CKD, how common it is, the risks connected to it, and why early detection, treatment, and teamwork are essential.

Acute Kidney Injury (AKI) is a sudden and temporary decline in kidney function that can occur over a short period of time, typically within a few hours or days. It is often caused by factors such as dehydration, infections, or exposure to certain medications or toxins. It is important to note that it is possible to have both AKI and CKD simultaneously. In such cases, once the AKI is addressed and resolved, the individual may see an improvement in their kidney function. However, this improvement does not mean that their CKD has been cured. They would still have CKD and need to continue monitoring and managing their kidney health, as the underlying chronic condition remains.

Prevalence and Impact of CKD

According to the Centers for Disease Control and Prevention

(CDC), approximately 14% of adults in the United States, or about 35.5 million people, are estimated to have CKD[1]. However, 9 out of 10 people with CKD are unaware of their condition, highlighting the importance of early detection and intervention (source: Centers for Disease Control and Prevention. (2023). Chronic Kidney Disease (CKD) National Facts. https://www.cdc.gov/kidneydisease/publications-resources/ckd-national-facts.html). Globally, the prevalence of CKD is also significant. A study published in Kidney International Supplements estimates that 10% of the world's population, or roughly 843.6 million people, are affected by CKD (source: Kovesdy, C. P. (2022). Epidemiology of chronic kidney disease: an update 2022. Kidney International Supplements, 12(1), 7-11. https://doi.org/10.1016/j.kisu.2021.11.003). It is the 12th leading cause of death worldwide and among the top 10 causes of death in Singapore, Greece, and Israel.

CKD is often referred to as a "silent" disease because it frequently progresses without noticeable symptoms until the later stages (commonly stages 4 & 5). This lack of overt symptoms makes early diagnosis challenging, leading to delayed treatment and a higher risk of severe complications. Consequently, CKD is recognized as a major public health issue and a leading cause of morbidity and mortality worldwide.

The economic burden of CKD is substantial, with healthcare systems around the world spending billions annually on CKD-related care. The costs associated with CKD encompass direct medical expenses, such as hospitalizations, dialysis, and medications, as well as indirect costs tied to lost productivity and disability. As the prevalence of CKD continues to climb, so does its economic impact, emphasizing the need for increased awareness, early detection, and effective management strategies.

The Progression of CKD

CKD is a progressive disease, meaning it worsens over time

as kidney function deteriorates. The progression of CKD is categorized into five stages based on the level of kidney function, as measured by the estimated glomerular filtration rate (eGFR). The eGFR is a calculation that estimates the volume of blood filtered by the kidneys per minute and is derived from blood tests measuring waste product levels, such as creatinine. Think of eGFR as your Kidney Function number – the higher it is, the better your kidneys are functioning.

The five stages of CKD are as follows:

- **Stage 1: eGFR 90 or Higher**

At this stage, kidney function is pretty much intact, and you might not even realize anything's amiss. Stage 1 is often asymptomatic and might simply be a result of the kidney's normal aging process. In most cases, it doesn't significantly impact one's lifestyle or overall health. If you are diagnosed at this stage, it's more of an alert to be vigilant about your kidney health than a cause for alarm.

- **Stage 2: eGFR 60-89**

When you hit Stage 2, the kidneys are still working well, but it's a wake-up call. This is when you need to scrutinize some of your lifestyle choices that could escalate the condition. It's time to address harmful habits like smoking, poor control of diabetes, or high blood pressure. Making some changes now could nip potential problems in the bud and preserve your kidney function for years to come.

- **Stage 3: eGFR 30-59**

By the time you reach Stage 3, it's crucial to put a heavy emphasis on a kidney-friendly, heart-healthy diet. Whole foods, low sodium, and balanced meals should become staples in your diet. Regular physical activity also becomes increasingly important. Monitoring your labs, as instructed by your healthcare team, will help adapt your treatment and dietary plans as necessary. In my experience, focusing on my diet and staying active are pivotal in slowing down the progression of kidney disease when at this stage.

- **Stage 4: eGFR 15-29**

Once you hit Stage 4, the need for careful management heightens exponentially. This is the stage where symptoms usually start to appear, and controlling blood pressure might become increasingly challenging. I'd strongly recommend learning about transplant options and even considering a preemptive transplant. Your diet will need to be more restrictive, possibly even supervised by a renal dietitian, to manage your symptoms and slow further decline of your kidney function.

- **Stage 5: eGFR Less Than 15**

Stage 5 is when your kidneys have almost stopped working, and you are approaching end-stage renal disease. At this stage, your healthcare team becomes your frontline defense. Effective symptom management and risk factor control are vital. Dialysis becomes a real possibility, and if a transplant isn't available, you'll need to start planning for it. When my eGFR was low, working closely with my healthcare team was indispensable. They helped me manage my symptoms and understand my treatment options, which included planning for the possibility of dialysis. Luckily for me I was able to make changes that improved my overall health and slowly moved me from Stage 5 back to Stage 3.

Navigating through the different stages of kidney disease can feel overwhelming, but the right knowledge and support can make a world of difference. Your healthcare team will be instrumental, but your own active role in managing your condition is equally important. And let's not forget the unparalleled strength that comes from a supportive family. My wife and children have been relentless in ensuring that I adhere to my lifestyle changes and treatment plans, making my journey with kidney disease far more bearable.

Individual Progression Rates

Kidney disease, much like many other conditions, does not follow a one-size-fits-all trajectory. The progression rate of this ailment can vary widely among individuals, emphasizing the inherent uniqueness of every patient's journey.

While some individuals may find their kidney function remains stable for decades without significant decline, others might experience a gradual deterioration, possibly transitioning from one stage of the disease to the next over the span of a decade or even longer. Contrarily, there are those who face a more rapid progression of kidney disease, with their kidney function declining at a considerably faster pace.

The medical landscape is continuously evolving, and with it, an array of treatment options and strategies are emerging that hold promise in slowing the progression of kidney disease. Renal dietary strategies, in particular, have been gaining traction and recognition for their role in managing and potentially decelerating the disease's advancement. Tailoring one's diet to the specific needs and restrictions of kidney disease can play a crucial role in maintaining better kidney function over time.

Tips to Slow Kidney Disease Progression:

- Regular Monitoring: Consistent check-ups and blood tests can help monitor kidney function, enabling timely interventions if any decline is observed.
- Follow Renal Diets: Adhering to a diet curated for kidney health can significantly reduce the strain on the kidneys. This might include managing protein intake, restricting certain minerals, and ensuring adequate hydration.
- Blood Pressure Management: High blood pressure can exacerbate kidney damage. Regular monitoring and management, either through lifestyle changes or

medication, is crucial.
- Blood Sugar Control: For those with diabetes, maintaining blood sugar levels within the recommended range can prevent further kidney damage.
- Limit Over-the-counter Medications: Some non-prescription drugs can be harmful to the kidneys. Always consult with a healthcare professional before taking any new medication.
- Stay Active: Regular exercise, tailored to one's capacity and health status, can help in overall health maintenance and manage conditions that might impact the kidneys.
- Avoid Smoking: Smoking can worsen kidney damage and further accelerate the progression of kidney disease.
- Limit Alcohol: Excessive alcohol can put additional strain on the kidneys. Moderation is key.
- Stay Educated: Keeping abreast with the latest research, treatments, and recommendations can empower patients and caregivers to make informed decisions.
- Avoid Self-Prescribing: It's common for those with kidney disease to look online and find recommendations for treatments that claim to improve kidney disease magically. Always, Always, Always review these with a doctor and never self-prescribe, thinking strangers on the Internet know better than medical science. The Internet has no end to the scams and dangerous treatment programs.

Common Symptoms of Kidney Disease

Symptoms Across Different Stages

Kidney disease often moves stealthily, frequently showing no symptoms until you hit the late stages. A common misconception is that symptoms become apparent early on. In reality, most people don't experience discernible symptoms until their eGFR goes below 30 or even as low as 15.

Recognizing the symptoms of late-stage kidney disease is essential for both patients and caregivers. At these advanced stages, symptoms are usually more prominent and may severely impact daily life. The following list outlines some of the common symptoms experienced at Stage 4 and Stage 5 of kidney disease.

Stage 4 Kidney Disease Symptoms

- Fatigue: Extreme tiredness even without much physical activity.
- Fluid Retention: Swelling in the extremities, particularly the legs, ankles, and feet.
- High Blood Pressure: Increasingly difficult to control despite medication.
- Urinary Changes: Frequent urination or the opposite, producing very little urine.
- Back or Side Pain: Pain in the kidney area, although not everyone experiences this.
- Changes in Taste: A metallic taste in the mouth is common.
- Nausea and Vomiting: Digestive issues may become frequent.
- Poor Appetite: Decrease in hunger levels.
- Brain Fog: Difficulty concentrating and remembering.
- Skin Issues: Dry and itchy skin.

Stage 5 Kidney Disease Symptoms

- Severe Fatigue: Almost constant tiredness, making daily activities hard to perform.

- Breathlessness: Difficulty in breathing, sometimes even when at rest.
- Frequent Hospitalizations: Increased susceptibility to infections.
- Muscle Cramps and Weakness: Particularly in the legs.
- Severe Nausea and Vomiting: Often unable to keep food down.
- Anemia: Very low energy levels due to fewer red blood cells.
- Persistent Headaches: Regular and often intense headaches.
- Shortness of Breath and Chest Pains: These symptoms are critical and should be reported immediately to a healthcare provider.
- Visual Disturbances: Issues like blurry vision.
- Irregular Heartbeat: Feelings of a fluttering or pounding heart.

For me, when my eGFR was as low as 13, I experienced a sudden onset of anemia, giving me extremely low energy levels. Headaches were consistent, and I had a persistent cough that seemed unshakable. Most challenging of all was the inability to keep food down. If you or your loved one experiences severe symptoms such as shortness of breath or chest pains, it's crucial to consult your healthcare team immediately. These could be signs of acute complications that require urgent intervention.

Kidney Vocabulary

Kidney disease comes with its own lexicon, and understanding this vocabulary can make your journey more navigable.

Nephrologist: This is a doctor who specializes in all things kidney. Think of them as your kidney guru. A Nephrologist will work with your family doctor in the treatment of your kidney disease.

eGFR/GFR: Standing for Estimated Glomerular Filtration Rate, this measures how well your kidneys are cleaning your blood. A simple way to think of this is the percentage of your kidney function remaining. This value is only an ESTIMATE and will naturally fluctuate. We want to focus on the trend and not a single value.

Creatinine: This is a waste product created naturally by your muscles that your kidneys should be filtering out of your blood. Creatinine is not bad for you, this it is only a marker used to estimate your kidney function. The more muscle mass you have, the higher your creatinine will be naturally. Avoid the common trap of trying to lower creatinine to improve your kidney health – it just doesn't work that way.

BUN (Blood Urea Nitrogen): Yet another waste product that the kidneys filter out. Elevated BUN levels indicate poor kidney function. Eating a diet rich in plant-based foods can be helpful in lowering your BUN.

Labs: These are the various tests that doctors perform to evaluate kidney function. Your doctor will let you know how often to get new labs.

Proteinuria: When there's too much protein in your urine, that's called proteinuria. It's a sign your kidneys aren't filtering as they should. Proteinuria is also a key indicator of future kidney problems. This can often be successfully managed with medication, such as an ACE or an ARB, along with a SLGT-2. From my experience, it is more important to focus on reducing protein in the urine than trying to increase your eGFR.

Anemia: A condition where the body doesn't have enough healthy red blood cells to deliver adequate oxygen to tissues, making the person feel tired or weak. One common cause of anemia, especially in kidney disease patients, is a deficiency of iron. The body needs iron to make red blood cells. To address this, doctors often recommend increasing iron intake, either through dietary changes or via supplements and injections, to boost the production of red blood cells and alleviate symptoms.

Renal Dietitian: This is a nutrition expert focused on helping people with kidney disease eat the right foods to support kidney function. I highly encourage all kidney patients to consult with a Renal Dietitian to assist in slowing the progression of kidney disease.

Renal Diet: The specially-designed eating plan for kidney disease patients. This is your kidney diet, which will be heart-healthy and full of plant-based foods.

ACE (Angiotensin-Converting Enzyme): A Common and very affordable type of blood pressure medication. Most kidney patients take either an ACE or an ARB.

ARB (Angiotensin II Receptor Blockers): A Common and very affordable type of blood pressure medication. Most kidney patients take either an ACE or an ARB.

SGLT-2 Inhibitor: A Common medication used with diabetics and kidney patients. It can lower blood sugar and help in reducing protein in the urine.

Importance of Early Detection and Proactivity in Treatment

Slowing Down the Disease

Early detection of kidney disease is akin to spotting a small leak in a dam. Address it right away, and you can avoid the impending flood. The sooner kidney disease is identified, the more effectively its progression can be slowed down. Standard tests for detection include measuring Blood Urea Nitrogen (BUN), Creatinine, and eGFR levels. Routine urine tests to check for proteinuria (protein in urine) can also be crucial for early diagnosis.

Being proactive about regular screenings is essential, especially for individuals who are at higher risk for kidney disease, such as those with diabetes, hypertension, or a family history of kidney-related issues. If you find that you are in the early stages of kidney disease (Stages 1 or 2), this is your alarm bell to kick bad habits, like smoking or consuming a diet rich in processed foods, to the curb. It's time to become fast friends with your healthcare team, including your nephrologist and renal dietitian, to tailor a management strategy suited for you.

Diet and Lifestyle Choices: The Pillars of Treatment

Now, let's not underestimate the power of diet and lifestyle changes. Oh boy, they're game-changers! A diet low in sodium, processed sugars, and saturated fats but rich in fruits, vegetables, and lean proteins can significantly slow the progression of kidney disease. I can personally vouch for the efficacy of diet in managing kidney disease—following a meticulously planned, renal-friendly diet has been one of the cornerstones of keeping me dialysis-free for over five years.

Physical activity is another factor not to be overlooked. Moderate exercise, under the supervision of healthcare providers, can not only improve overall well-being but also help in better management of blood pressure and blood sugar levels—two key players in kidney health.

The Support of Loved Ones: My Personal Pillar

My journey with kidney disease has not been a solo venture. My wife and children have been invaluable caregivers, filling roles that range from emotional support to diet planning. Their resilience and love have been foundational in empowering me to make healthier choices every day. Knowing that I am not alone on this trek has been a significant motivational factor in adhering to lifestyle modifications.

The Kidney-Heart Connection: A Two-Way Street

One aspect of kidney disease that often slides under the radar is its symbiotic relationship with heart health. Kidney disease can be both a cause and a consequence of cardiovascular diseases. Elevated levels of toxins in the blood due to reduced kidney function can strain the heart and lead to conditions like hypertension and heart failure.

Conversely, heart conditions can compromise kidney function by reducing blood flow to the kidneys. It's a bit of a chicken-and-egg scenario, which makes it all the more important to focus on a heart-healthy lifestyle. Dietary choices beneficial for the kidneys, like reducing salt and fat intake, naturally align with a heart-healthy approach. Medications like ACE inhibitors or ARBs often serve dual roles in managing both heart and kidney conditions.

By embracing early detection and a proactive treatment approach, coupled with unwavering support from loved ones, it's entirely possible to slow down the progression of kidney disease and maintain an uplifting quality of life. Remember, kidney disease is not a death sentence; it's a life-altering condition that can be managed effectively with the right tools and mindset.

THE EMOTIONAL ROLLERCOASTER

If there's one thing that's certain about a kidney disease diagnosis, it's that the emotional landscape will shift dramatically. Initially, a torrent of varied feelings—shock, disbelief, numbness—will engulf the individual. The diagnosis may feel like a metaphorical black hole, sucking in hope and leaving an emotional void.

Shortly after diagnosis, an avalanche of information follows. Medical terms like eGFR, creatinine levels, and nephrologist appointments may suddenly become part of daily discussions. The complexity of the disease necessitates learning an almost new language, turning patients and caregivers into amateur linguists, scrambling to understand the healthcare lexicon.

In this journey, both the diagnosed individual and the caregiver face the harsh reality that kidney disease is a chronic condition with no outright cure. The permanence of this situation is daunting. It's like getting onto a train with an unknown destination, staring out of the window as familiar landmarks recede into the distance.

Given the long-term nature of the disease, dietary and lifestyle adjustments become inescapable. What once were simple choices—like what to eat for dinner—become critical decisions affecting kidney function. This transforms regular activities into constant reminders of the illness, like persistent post-it notes on the refrigerator door of life.

Medications become a relentless regimen to adhere to. Each

pill, each dosage, becomes a cog in the machine of health maintenance. A missed pill isn't just a forgotten task; it's a crack in the fortress built to combat kidney deterioration. This adds another layer to the emotional complexity, as guilt and self-blame may ensue for any slip-ups.

Given the multifaceted nature of managing kidney disease, it's no surprise that a person's motivation levels will waver. It is not uncommon for initial bursts of proactive behavior to gradually fizzle out. Caregivers will find that maintaining a constant level of motivation in their loved one requires a delicate balancing act, like a tightrope walker wobbling between lapses and leaps of willpower.

Foundations of Support: How to Truly Be There for Your Loved One

Supporting someone with kidney disease requires a multifaceted approach that goes far beyond just being a shoulder to cry on. If you are reading this book, you are already taking a significant stride in becoming an informed and therefore effective caregiver—a beacon in the confusing landscape of kidney disease.

Your role begins with self-education. Understanding every nuance of Chronic Kidney Disease (CKD) allows you to be not just emotionally supportive but also practically helpful. This means learning about the condition's medical intricacies, medication protocols, and research-backed dietary adjustments.

Active listening is not just a conversational virtue; it's an emotional lifesaver in the kidney disease journey. When your loved one wants to express their fears, frustrations, or even fleeting moments of optimism, your attentive listening provides them an invaluable emotional outlet.

It's important to remember that empathy doesn't mean absorbing all of the diagnosed individual's emotional stress. Establishing clear emotional boundaries is crucial. You are a companion in their journey, not an emotional storage unit. Strive to provide emotional availability while also safeguarding your emotional well-being.

Your support will manifest in diverse ways. Sometimes, it could be in seemingly trivial tasks like ensuring a continuous stock of kidney-friendly foods at home, or more significantly, accompanying them to medical appointments and actively participating in conversations with healthcare providers.

Initial Coping Mechanisms: Navigating Early Responses and Reactions

Ah, coping mechanisms—the psychological lifejackets people clutch onto when tossed into the turbulent waters of a chronic disease diagnosis. The initial stage following a diagnosis of kidney disease often leads individuals into a labyrinth of emotional responses and coping strategies. To describe it as a rollercoaster would be an understatement; it's more like a labyrinthine maze with its twists, turns, and occasional dead-ends.

The first coping mechanism that often comes into play is denial, the mental shield that buffers people from the immediate impact of reality. This is not just a river in Egypt, folks! Denial can manifest in different ways: minimizing the severity of the disease, neglecting medication, or even avoiding follow-up appointments with healthcare providers. As a caregiver, you might find it frustrating, but understand that denial is a natural psychological response. The key is not to clash head-on with it but gently guide your loved one towards acceptance and action.

Now, swinging to the other end of the spectrum, we have what I call the "Overzealous Transformer." This individual goes full throttle into lifestyle changes. We're talking Spartan diets, marathon-like exercise sessions, and perhaps even a deep dive into alternative treatments, often without sufficient research or professional guidance. While the enthusiasm is admirable, the approach can be hazardous. The body, especially one dealing with kidney disease, needs time to adjust to changes. Rapid shifts can lead to other medical issues or exacerbate existing ones. As a caregiver, your role is to encourage moderation and consultation with healthcare providers.

Resourcefulness is another coping mechanism that often appears. Your loved one may suddenly become a Google scholar, diving into forums, medical papers, and even snake oil salesmen disguised as miracle cure websites. While being informed is crucial, the danger lies in the credibility of the sources consulted. Your role? Be the beacon of credible information. Guide them to legitimate sources like scholarly articles, official health websites, and advice from medical professionals. Make sure that the information they are absorbing is accurate and beneficial.

Documentation can serve as a highly effective coping strategy. In the sea of emotional chaos, maintaining a log or journal can act as an anchor. Some individuals find comfort in recording their symptoms, food intake, emotional states, and medical readings. This not only helps in tracking disease progression but also provides a valuable resource for healthcare providers. As a caregiver, you can facilitate this by perhaps providing a journal or introducing them to health tracking apps. Your active involvement demonstrates emotional support and practical assistance.

Another coping mechanism worth mentioning is withdrawal or isolation. Facing a chronic disease can sometimes feel like carrying a heavy, invisible backpack. Some people feel so weighed down that they pull away from social activities, avoid discussions about their condition, or even isolate themselves from loved ones. While it's important to respect their need for space, total isolation is unhealthy. Encourage them to stay connected with family and friends and perhaps join a support group. Your role here is nuanced; it's about respecting their need for solitude while also emphasizing the importance of social support for emotional well-being.

So, how do you, the caregiver, navigate this myriad of coping mechanisms? First and foremost, look after yourself. You can't pour from an empty cup. Emotional fatigue is real, and you're not immune. Maintain your circle of support among friends, family, or caregiver support groups. Prioritize activities that recharge your emotional and physical energy. This self-care equips you to better support your loved one through their emotional labyrinth.

In essence, the early stages of coping with a kidney disease diagnosis are a complex web of emotional reactions and actions. Your role as a caregiver is far from one-dimensional. You're part-coach, part-guide, and part-therapist. Navigating initial coping mechanisms requires a nuanced understanding of human psychology, a sprinkle of medical knowledge, a dash of emotional intelligence, and an enormous amount of patience. This is not a sprint; it's a marathon. And each moment of support and understanding you provide helps in laying the foundation for the long journey ahead.

Shifting Sands: Family Dynamics in the Wake of Chronic Illness

A chronic illness like kidney disease does more than just affect the individual; it fundamentally alters the family unit's dynamics. Spouses, children, and even extended family are pulled into the vortex of change that a chronic condition inevitably brings about.

Roles within the family undergo transformation. If the diagnosed person was a primary caretaker or the main breadwinner, the shift in these roles can be jarring. It often leads to an unplanned, immediate restructuring of household responsibilities. Children may suddenly find themselves taking on adult-like responsibilities, causing an accelerated loss of innocence.

Emotions among family members can also become volatile. While the primary focus is understandably on the diagnosed individual, other family members may experience feelings of neglect. This could lead to resentment, triggering internal conflicts that add another layer of complexity to an already challenging situation.

Relationships with friends and extended family may also see a change. While some may offer incredible support, others may distance themselves, either due to discomfort or a lack of understanding of how to help. Such fluctuations in social support can be disheartening but are an unfortunate reality.

Recognizing these changes and addressing them through open communication is critical. Scheduled family meetings or professional counseling can serve as platforms for everyone to express their concerns, fears, and expectations. This collective approach promotes a more harmonious living environment, making the challenging journey ahead slightly less daunting for everyone involved.

NAVIGATING DIETARY CHANGES AS A FAMILY

Navigating the path of kidney health often leads to significant shifts in dietary choices, presenting challenges and learning opportunities for both the individual diagnosed and their family. Diet plays an instrumental role in managing kidney disease, with certain modifications offering the potential to slow its progression. This chapter delves deep into understanding the renal diet's intricacies and its paramount importance. For caregivers and loved ones, this chapter serves as a guiding light, emphasizing the collective journey of adjusting to these dietary changes. By exploring this journey together, families can foster a supportive environment, ensuring that nutritional choices become a collaborative, informed, and even enjoyable endeavor.

The Renal Diet

When a family member gets diagnosed with kidney disease, there is often a whirlwind of emotions followed by a tornado of information—medications, treatments, and yes, the all-important renal diet. Understanding the renal diet is like decoding an intricate puzzle; it's complex but crucial for managing kidney disease. What you eat significantly impacts your kidney function, and the renal diet is designed to lighten the load on these essential organs.

A renal diet is a dietary plan tailored to meet the unique needs of someone with kidney disease. It usually involves restrictions on protein, phosphorus, sodium, and eventually potassium. But do not despair; it's not about a list of 'no-nos,' but more about balance and portion control. The renal diet plays a pivotal role in slowing the progression of kidney disease and can help in managing symptoms more effectively.

The phrase 'one size fits all' might work for scarves or hats, but certainly not for a renal diet. The body is not a machine with standard specifications; it's a complex, biological entity. That's why it is crucial to have a renal diet customized to your loved one's specific needs. This customization typically depends on the stage of kidney disease, the presence of other medical conditions like diabetes, and the latest lab results. The diet may evolve over time as the kidney function changes. A benefit of an individualized diet is that focus is on portion control rather than a list of foods not to eat. Foods that are less kidney-friendly, such as pizza, can still be enjoyed from time to time, but in smaller portion sizes (perhaps a single slice instead of 3).

Enter the role of a Renal Dietitian—your personalized guide in this dietary journey. A Renal Dietitian has specialized training in managing diet for kidney diseases. They can interpret lab results, assess nutritional needs, and develop an individualized dietary plan. If you think of the renal diet as a unique language, consider the dietitian as your personal linguist, interpreting the complexities for you.

Plant-based diets can be a game-changer in this scenario. They are naturally lower in sodium and phosphorus and can be less taxing on the kidneys. According to a study in the American Journal of Kidney Disease, plant-based diets are associated with a lower risk of chronic kidney disease. Not to mention, they have an additional slew of benefits like lower cholesterol levels, improved blood sugar control, and better weight management. (source: Joshi, S., McMacken, M., & Kalantar-

Zadeh, K. (2021). Plant-Based Diets for Kidney Disease: A Guide for Clinicians. American journal of kidney diseases : the official journal of the National Kidney Foundation, 77(2), 287–296. https://doi.org/10.1053/j.ajkd.2020.10.003)

However, 'plant-based' does not mean vegetarian or vegan. It just emphasizes fruits, vegetables, legumes, and whole grains. Meat can still find a place on the plate but in moderation and lean cuts. Some people get creative and use plant-based meat substitutes for a meaty texture without the added animal protein.

Being the caregiver, you're often the one planning meals, grocery shopping, and even cooking. So your understanding of the renal diet is not just essential, it's transformative for your loved one's health journey. In your role, you also serve as a motivator encouraging your family member to stick to the diet, reminding them it's not a list of "don'ts" but a creative challenge in eating right.

Your involvement creates a ripple effect. By embracing the renal diet, you're subtly encouraging the whole family to eat healthier. This not only supports your loved one with kidney disease but also sets a healthy dining table, benefiting everyone involved.

You might encounter resistance from your loved one initially. Changing lifelong eating habits is not easy, and the fear of missing out on favorite foods can lead to stress. Here is where you can be a source of creative solutions. Explore kidney-friendly recipes together, experiment with spices to replace salt, or find joy in discovering new vegetables and fruits that fit into the renal diet.

The renal diet can seem daunting at first glance, but once you dive in, it becomes a powerful tool. It's not about deprivation; it's about making smarter choices. It's not a diet in the conventional sense, but more of a lifestyle change. Your role as a caregiver in navigating this change cannot be overstated.

Grocery Shopping 101

Ah, the art of grocery shopping. Gone are the days when you could just pick anything off the shelf. With kidney disease in the picture, grocery shopping turns into a strategic mission. You become the gatekeeper of nutrition, tasked with bringing home foods that are tasty and kidney-friendly.

Start by bidding farewell to processed foods that are high in sodium. Checking food labels becomes your new best friend. Sodium sneaks its way into seemingly harmless foods like canned soups, frozen dinners, and even some breakfast cereals. Ideally, aim for foods with less than 140 mg of sodium per serving. Many doctors recommend a diet with 2000 mg or less of sodium per day.

Potassium is a bit of a tricky customer. It's essential for heart health, but too much of a good thing can be harmful. In the early stages of kidney disease, normal potassium levels are usually encouraged. However, as your loved one progresses to stage 4 or 5, potassium levels may need to be monitored more carefully, and a reduction in high-potassium foods may become necessary.

Phosphorus is another nutrient you should keep an eye on. It's found naturally in many foods, but when it comes to processed items, phosphorus often appears as an additive. High phosphorus levels can cause complications like bone disorders in kidney patients. You can spot phosphorus additives on food labels as phrases like "PHOS" such as 'calcium phosphate.'

Fresh fruits and vegetables should be a staple in your grocery list, but even here, choices matter. Opt for low-potassium choices like apples, berries, and grapes and avoid high-potassium fruits like bananas, oranges, and melons. When it comes to vegetables, leafy greens are your best bet. However, some like spinach and Swiss chard are high in potassium, so be selective.

Grains and cereals are generally good, especially whole grains like whole-wheat bread and brown rice. However, whole grains are also higher in phosphorus and potassium compared to their refined counterparts. So, the choice between whole and refined grains might depend on your loved one's specific dietary needs.

Dairy and dairy alternatives are also an area where you need to tread carefully. Regular dairy is high in phosphorus, so you might need to switch to non-dairy alternatives like almond milk or rice milk. But remember to check for added phosphates.

As for meats, go lean. Fish, chicken, and turkey are better options compared to red meats. However, fish can be high in phosphorus, so portion control is key.

Staying Hydrated: Quenching Thirst the Kidney-Friendly Way

The importance of hydration cannot be overstressed, especially for those with kidney disease. Our kidneys play a pivotal role in fluid management, ensuring the right balance for our body's optimal functioning. But, with kidney disease, the typical "rules" of hydration can shift, presenting a new set of considerations. If you're caring for a loved one with kidney disease, understanding these nuances is crucial.

Water remains the gold standard for hydration. It's pure, refreshing, and free from additives or extra calories. It helps flush out toxins and supports overall kidney health. If plain water seems uninteresting, a splash of lemon or a sprig of mint can add a hint of natural flavor, making it more palatable. For those chilly evenings, herbal teas are a delightful alternative. They're not only warm and comforting but also present an opportunity to introduce various flavors without any adverse effects on the kidneys.

Coffee lovers, rejoice! Yes, coffee can be a part of the renal diet. But, it's essential to be mindful of the extras. Those dollops of cream, flavored syrups, or spoonfuls of sugar can quickly turn a kidney-friendly drink into a not-so-friendly one. Especially the phosphorus commonly found in commercial additives. So, while that occasional latte or cappuccino can still be enjoyed, it's essential to keep tabs on the added ingredients.

Sodas, particularly dark-colored ones, are a tricky territory. These often come loaded with sugars, artificial flavors, and, notably, phosphorus additives, which can be hard on compromised kidneys. As a caregiver, guiding your loved one towards healthier choices and away from these potential pitfalls is vital. Besides, making healthier beverage choices yourself can set a positive example, making the transition smoother.

It's a common myth that more fluids equals healthier kidneys. While hydration is crucial, overhydration can strain kidneys, especially if their function is already compromised. This is where the healthcare team steps in. They can provide guidelines on the appropriate daily fluid intake based on the patient's specific condition and needs. These guidelines ensure that the body receives adequate hydration without overwhelming the kidneys.

A challenge that might arise as kidney disease progresses is fluid restriction. When kidney function diminishes significantly, they may struggle to handle excessive fluid intake. In such cases, a doctor might recommend a daily limit on fluid intake. If this occurs, it's essential to be supportive and help your loved one stick to these guidelines, ensuring they don't feel deprived.

An excellent way to monitor fluid intake is to use a designated jug or bottle for the day. Fill it to the prescribed limit each morning and use only this container throughout the day. It provides a clear visual cue and helps in pacing the intake.

Family Meals: Crafting Kidney-Friendly and Low-Sodium Feasts

The dining table can either be a battlefield or a peace zone when dealing with dietary restrictions. Many families have traditions and comfort foods that they cherish, and the thought of giving them up can feel like losing a part of your identity. But the good news? Adaptation is the name of the game. You don't have to give up family favorites; you just need to modify them to make them kidney-friendly.

First things first, let's talk about salt. Sodium is a huge no-no in a renal diet, but that doesn't mean your foods have to be bland. Get creative with your spices. Swap out table salt for fresh herbs like parsley, basil, or chives to add flavor. A dash of lemon juice or a sprinkle of pepper can also elevate a dish without the sodium. Consider salt-free seasoning blends that are widely available in grocery stores; just be sure to read the labels to ensure they are truly sodium-free. Here are some helpful seasoning combos I often use:

- Asparagus: Garlic, Lemon Juice, Onion, Vinegar
- Beef: Basil, Bay Leaf, Chilis, Coriander, Garlic, Green Pepper, Marjoram, Mushrooms, Mustard, Nutmeg, Onion, Oregano, Parsley, Pepper, Safe, Tarragon, Thyme
- Bread: Anise, Basil, Caraway, Cardamom, Cinnamon, Cloves, Cumin, Dill, Lemon Peel, Poppy Seeds, Saffron, Sesame Seeds
- Broccoli: Lemon Juice, Garlic
- Cheese: Caraway, Celery Seed, Chervil, Chives, Curry, Dill, Garlic, Horseradish, Lemon Peel, Mustard, Nutmeg, Parsley, Pepper, Sage
- Chicken: Allspice, Basil, Bay Leaf, Cinnamon, Curry, Dill, Garlic, Ginger, Lime, Lemon, Marjoram, Mushrooms, Oregano, Paprika, Parsley, Poultry Seasoning, Saffron, Sage, Tarragon, Thyme
- Cucumbers: Chives, Dill, Garlic, Onion, Vinegar
- Eggs: Basil, Chervil, Chives, Curry, Dill, Fennel, Ginger, Paprika, Parsley, Pepper, Sage, Tarragon
- Fish: Basil, Bay Leaf, Chives, Curry, Dill, Fennel, Garlic, Ginger, Lemon, Mustard, Paprika, Parsley, Tarragon

- Fruit: Allspice, Anise, Cardamom, Cinnamon, Cloves, Coriander, Ginger, Mint, Nutmeg
- Green Beans: Dill, Lemon Juice, Nutmeg, Marjoram
- Greens: Onion, Pepper, Vinegar
- Lamb: Basil, Bay Leaf, Cinnamon, Coriander, Cumin, Curry, Dill, Garlic, Mint, Parsley, Pineapple, Rosemary, Tarragon, Thyme
- Pasta: Basil, Caraway Seed, Garlic, Oregano, Poppy Seed
- Peas: Green Pepper, Mint, Parsley, Onion, Fresh Mushrooms
- Pork: Apple, Applesauce, Garlic, Onion, Sage
- Potatoes: Green Pepper, Mace, Onion, Paprika, Parsley
- Rice: Chives, Green Pepper, Saffron, Onion
- Salad Dressings: Basil, Chives, Dill, Fennel, Garlic, Horseradish, Mustard, Oregano, Paprika, Parsley, Saffron, Tarragon
- Salads: Basil, Chives, Dill, Garlic, Lemon, Mint, Oregano, Parsley, Tarragon
- Salt Substitutes: Allspice, Basil, Bay Leaf, Caraway, Cardamom, Curry, Dash, Dill, Ginger, Marjoram, Rosemary, Thyme, Safe, Tarragon
- Soups (Homemade): Basil, Bay Leaf, Chervil, Chilis, Chives, Cumin, Dill, Fennel, Garlic, Parsley, Pepper, Rosemary, Sage, Thyme
- Squash: Cinnamon, Nutmeg, Mace, Ginger
- Sweets: Allspice, Anise, Cardamom, Cinnamon, Cloves, Fennel, Lemon Peel, Ginger, Mace, Nutmeg, Mint
- Tomatoes: Basil, Marjoram, Onion, Oregano,
- Veal: Apricot, Cinnamon, Cloves, Ginger

Adapting recipes often involve substitutions. For example, if a recipe calls for regular pasta, consider switching to whole grain pasta for added fiber and nutrients. Just keep in mind that whole grains are higher in phosphorus, so portion control is key. If dairy is in the mix, you might want to opt for non-dairy alternatives like almond milk or rice milk, which are lower in phosphorus. Again, be cautious of additives.

Speaking of additives, let's dive into sauces and gravies. They often contain hidden sodium and phosphorus. Consider making your own at home where you control the ingredients. A tomato sauce made from fresh tomatoes, herbs, and a splash of olive oil can be both delicious and kidney-friendly. The same goes for gravy; using a low-sodium broth and avoiding processed thickeners can make a world of difference.

When it comes to protein, think beyond the traditional. Fish like salmon and tuna are excellent choices as they provide essential omega-3 fatty acids. However, it's good to keep portion sizes in check as fish can also be high in phosphorus. Plant-based proteins like lentils and chickpeas are also great options but remember to consult with your renal dietitian as they contain higher amounts of potassium and phosphorus.

Vegetables are your best friends but choose wisely. Low-potassium options like cauliflower, bell peppers, and green beans are good choices. You can even get creative and use cauliflower as a substitute for mashed potatoes or pizza crust. It's all about getting inventive in the kitchen.

Fruits can be a delicious and healthy addition to meals but stick to low-potassium options like apples, blueberries, and strawberries. Fresh fruit is often better than dried fruit or fruit juices, which can be high in sugar and other additives. Include them in desserts or as a natural sweetener to dishes.

Healthy oils like olive oil or avocado oil are good for cooking and for dressings. They contain heart-healthy fats that can also help manage cholesterol levels, a bonus when dealing with kidney disease, which often has coexisting conditions like hypertension or heart issues.

Nuts and seeds like almonds and chia seeds can be added to dishes for crunch and nutrition. However, they are also high in phosphorus and potassium, so portion control is key. A small sprinkle can go a long way in adding texture and flavor.

Meal planning is another critical component. Plan your week in advance, paying close attention to balancing nutrients across meals. This not only makes grocery shopping easier but also helps you stick to a renal-friendly diet. Plus, meal planning is a great activity to do together as a family, as everyone can chip in with their preferences and ideas.

Last but not least, remember that you're setting an example. By taking the time to adapt recipes and make them kidney-friendly, you're showing how much you care, not just about the family member with kidney disease but for the well-being of everyone at the table. Your proactive role in maintaining a kidney-friendly kitchen serves as a role model, teaching valuable lessons about health and adaptability to the younger members of the family.

Dining Out: Guiding Your Loved One Through Restaurant Choices

Ah, the delight of a restaurant meal! It's often seen as a break from the norm, a time to enjoy the company of family and friends. However, when you're a caregiver for someone with kidney disease, the idea of dining out might initially seem daunting. Fear not! With a bit of pre-planning and strategic thinking, you can help your loved one enjoy a meal out without compromising their kidney health.

Firstly, embrace the gift of technology. Most restaurants today have their menus available online, and this is a fantastic tool at your disposal. Before heading out, review the menu with your loved one. You can identify potential dishes that align well with their renal diet, enabling them to make a smart, kidney-friendly selection. It can remove the stress of in-the-moment decision-making and allows both of you to focus more on the experience rather than fretting over the food.

Remember, communication is key. When you're ordering, don't hesitate to discuss any necessary dietary modifications with the server or chef. From asking for dressings on the side to requesting a preferred cooking method, restaurants are generally accommodating when it comes to special dietary needs. Helping your loved one vocalize these needs not only ensures a better meal for them but also serves as an educational moment.

Being proactive about sides and sauces can be a game-changer. Most sauces and dressings are sodium traps, and we don't need those. Ask for them on the side, so your loved one can manage how much to use. This level of control is empowering and aligns well with maintaining a renal-friendly diet.

Selecting the right main course and side dishes is crucial. Advise your loved one to opt for lean proteins that are grilled or baked instead of fried or breaded. Side options like steamed vegetables can be a safer bet compared to fries or rice pilaf, which often contain hidden sodium or phosphorus.

Flavor should never be a compromise, even with dietary restrictions. Bringing along a small container of kidney-safe herbs or seasonings can be a wonderful way to add some personalized flavor to a meal. A sprinkle of dried herbs or a squeeze of fresh lemon juice can elevate a dish while keeping it within the safety zone of a renal diet.

Portion control is often overlooked but incredibly important. Restaurant portions can be generous, and while that's generally a good thing, it's not ideal for someone on a renal diet. Consider sharing dishes or taking half of it home for another meal. This strategy helps keep meal portions in check and provides an extra meal for later—a double win!

Remember, hydration matters, even on a night out. While the beverage menu might be tempting, sticking to water or herbal teas is usually the safest bet. Help your loved one make a wise choice that won't lead to additional concerns about fluid restrictions or additives.

What about the dessert menu? It's not off-limits, but it does require some scrutiny. A fruit-based dessert, like a sorbet or fruit salad, can often satisfy the sweet tooth without going overboard on sugar or other additives. Again, sharing a dessert can offer a taste without causing a dietary derailment.

In summary, dining out with your loved one who has kidney disease is not only feasible but can also be an enjoyable, stress-free experience. It just requires a bit of planning and strategic choice-making. This preparation not only ensures a meal that aligns with their kidney health but also offers a much-needed sense of normality and enjoyment. So go ahead, make that reservation, and relish the rich experience of dining out! After all, taking care of someone doesn't mean depriving them or yourself of life's little joys. It's about finding a way to make it work for everyone involved. Cheers to finding that balance!

FAMILY WORKOUTS FOR KIDNEY HEALTH

Physical activity plays a pivotal role in managing and potentially slowing the progression of kidney disease. For caregivers and families, fostering an environment that promotes regular workouts and shared activities can be invaluable. This chapter provides a holistic view of integrating exercise into the daily routine, emphasizing its significance and outlining strategies tailored for those with kidney conditions. Through joint family efforts, exercise can become not just a therapeutic tool, but also a bonding experience, fostering closer relationships and healthier outcomes.

Why Exercise Matters

Exercise, often deemed a cornerstone of general health, takes on an even more pivotal role for individuals grappling with kidney disease. For caregivers, understanding the profound implications of incorporating regular physical activity into a loved one's routine can be a game-changer in their kidney disease journey.Moreover, exercise enhances muscle strength and endurance. This is particularly significant for those with kidney disease, as they often grapple with fatigue and weakness. Regular workouts can help combat these symptoms, lending them more energy and vitality in daily activities. It's not just about physical prowess but also about reclaiming the joy in everyday tasks.

Unpacking the Physical Advantages:

The merits of exercise in the context of kidney disease are multifarious and undeniable:

- Strengthening Muscle Function: Regular physical activity acts as a bulwark against muscle atrophy, often associated with kidney disease. It aids in preserving and often amplifying muscle strength, ensuring tasks of daily living are accomplished with ease and independence.
- Heart and Vascular Health: Cardiovascular complications often cast a long shadow on kidney disease patients. Embracing a structured exercise regimen bolsters heart health, fortifies vascular walls, and maintains optimal blood pressure levels, thus mitigating potential cardiac concerns.
- Promoting Bone Vitality: The specter of reduced bone density looms large for many with kidney disease. Engaging in weight-bearing exercises, from brisk walking to resistance training, can enhance bone mineral density, warding off fractures and brittleness.
- Optimal Weight Management: With kidney disease, maintaining a balanced weight becomes even more crucial. Exercise serves as a dual-edged sword, aiding in weight loss and staving off unwanted weight gain, thereby alleviating undue strain on the kidneys.
- Combating Anemia: Enhanced circulation, a product of regular exercise, can play a role in the better distribution of oxygen-carrying red blood cells, potentially providing relief from the fatigue and lethargy accompanying anemia, a frequent companion of kidney disease.

The Psychological and Emotional Efficacy:
Beyond the undeniable physical dividends, exercise bestows a wealth of emotional and psychological boons:

- Elevated Mental State: The act of moving, of challenging one's limits, triggers the release of endorphins – nature's mood elevators. For someone grappling with kidney disease, this can provide respite from the occasional mental clouds of despair or anxiety.
- Restorative Sleep: The link between physical activity and sleep quality is well-documented. For kidney patients, a night of restful sleep can rejuvenate both body and mind, preparing them for the day ahead.
- Boosting Self-worth: Progress, no matter how incremental, when charted through exercise milestones, can ignite a sense of achievement and bolster self-esteem. This often translates to a more positive outlook on life and its challenges.

My Personal Testament:
When I was first diagnosed, the shadow of anemia cast a pall over my everyday life. The mere act of walking from the bed to the bathroom felt Herculean. But, with the relentless encouragement and unwavering support of my family, I pushed the boundaries of what I thought possible. Initial, seemingly insurmountable challenges like reaching the mailbox transformed into triumphs. Over time, those short distances evolved into longer treks, culminating in a mile-long walk around the neighborhood. Each step became a testament to resilience, each milestone a beacon of hope. This exercise journey was not just about physical recovery; it was a symbolic march towards reclaiming life, illustrating that kidney disease was a chapter, not the entirety of the narrative.

Tracking Progress

To truly harness the benefits of exercise, especially for someone with kidney disease, it is essential not only to commit to a regimen but also to systematically track its effects. Monitoring progress paints a comprehensive picture of health and provides tangible evidence of improvement, acting as a source of motivation and validation for the effort invested.

1. Blood Pressure Monitoring:
For kidney patients, maintaining optimal blood pressure is pivotal.

- Why Track: Elevated blood pressure levels can exacerbate kidney complications. Regular monitoring allows timely interventions and medication adjustments, if necessary.
- How to Track: Invest in a home blood pressure monitor. Taking daily readings, preferably at the same time each day, can give insights into any fluctuations and patterns.

2. Weight Management:
Keeping an eye on weight is crucial, especially when exercise is introduced.

- Why Track: Weight changes can offer insights into fluid retention, dietary effects, and the impact of the exercise routine.
- How to Track: Regular weigh-ins, preferably at the same time of day using a calibrated scale, can provide consistent data. Weekly or bi-weekly tracking can capture meaningful changes.

3. Endurance Levels:
Endurance is an excellent barometer for cardiovascular health and overall fitness.

- Why Track: Increases in endurance can indicate improved heart health, lung capacity, and muscle strength.
- How to Track: Setting periodic goals, such as walking a certain distance or engaging in an activity for a

set duration, and noting the time taken or the ease with which these are achieved can offer insights into endurance progress.

4. Keeping a Journal:
A detailed exercise journal can be the cornerstone of tracking.

- Why Track: A journal provides a holistic view of exercise routines, feelings, challenges faced, and milestones achieved.
- How to Track: Dedicate a few minutes post-exercise to jot down the activity undertaken, its duration, intensity, and any bodily responses like fatigue or soreness. Over time, this log can reflect progress and areas that need attention.

5. Tracking Flexibility and Strength:
Strength and flexibility exercises, though subtle, can bring about significant changes.

- Why Track: Improved flexibility can enhance joint health and reduce the risk of injuries. Strength training, on the other hand, can bolster muscle mass and overall functional fitness.
- How to Track: Set periodic benchmarks. For flexibility, it could be reaching toes or stretching arms to a certain point. For strength, it might be the number of repetitions of a particular exercise or the weight lifted.

6. Technology and Apps:
Leverage technology to streamline tracking.

- Why Track: Digital tools offer a convenient and organized way to keep track of various metrics and often provide graphical representations of progress.
- How to Track: Numerous fitness and health tracking apps are available that can log exercise routines, blood pressure readings, weight changes, and more. These

apps often come with reminders, ensuring consistent data entry.

Safety First

Safety, undoubtedly, is paramount. While exercise boasts numerous benefits, diving in without precautions can be counterproductive, especially for kidney patients.

For those on dialysis, the placement of the catheter or fistula must be considered. Engaging in exercises that put undue pressure or strain on these areas should be avoided. Swimming, though an excellent aerobic exercise, may be off-limits for some dialysis patients due to potential infection risks through the catheter site. However, walking, cycling, or gentle yoga can be safe alternatives.

Dehydration is another concern. Kidney patients, especially those on a fluid restriction, should be cautious about not over-exerting to the point of excessive sweating. It's vital to balance fluid intake with the amount lost during exercise. This doesn't mean they should shy away from physical activity, but hydration levels should be monitored closely.

Bone health is crucial. Some kidney patients might have weakened bones due to the disease or medications. Weight-bearing exercises can help strengthen bones, but it's essential to start slow and potentially avoid high-impact activities that might risk fractures.

Muscle cramping, a frequent complaint among kidney patients, can be exacerbated by certain exercises. Stretching routines and adequate hydration can help in preventing or alleviating these cramps.

Remember, everyone is different. What works for one patient might not work for another. Regular consultation with healthcare professionals before starting or modifying any exercise regimen is essential. They can provide tailored advice, keeping in mind the specific needs and challenges of the patient.

Lastly, as a caregiver, it's your role to ensure that exercises are performed in a safe environment, free from hazards like slippery floors or obstacles. Offering support, both emotionally and physically, can make the exercise journey smoother and safer for your loved one.

Fun Activities

Exercise is undoubtedly beneficial for kidney patients, but let's face it: the word "workout" can sound dreary to many. So, how do we shift the perspective from a laborious task to a fun-filled activity? Making workouts enjoyable not only boosts adherence but also creates lasting memories for both the patient and the caregiver. Here are some tips to infuse joy into the exercise regimen:

- Variety is the Spice of Life: The same routine can quickly become monotonous. Introducing variety keeps things fresh and interesting. For instance, if walking is the primary exercise, consider occasionally swapping it with dancing or a fun aerobics session. Every few weeks, introducing a new form of exercise can keep the enthusiasm alive. As a caregiver, you can join in, making it a delightful duo activity.
- Outdoor Adventures: Nature has a therapeutic touch. Shifting exercises outdoors can be invigorating. Whether it's practicing yoga in a park, cycling along scenic routes, or hiking on beginner trails, the beauty of nature can make workouts feel less like a chore. The fresh air, chirping of birds, and the serene environment can elevate the mood, making the entire experience pleasant.
- Group Activities: There's strength in numbers. Engaging in group activities can be a game-changer. Joining a local exercise group or a dance class can

introduce social interactions, making workouts more enjoyable. Sharing stories, progress, and challenges with fellow participants can provide mutual motivation. As a caregiver, fostering such community interactions can be beneficial for your loved one's mental well-being.
- Gamify the Process: Incorporate elements of play. Thanks to technology, there are numerous fitness apps and gadgets that turn exercises into games. Whether it's achieving daily step targets, completing virtual races, or even interactive video games that require physical movement, such tools can make workouts thrilling. Celebrate the small victories, whether it's reaching a certain number of steps or mastering a dance move.
- Music and Rhythms: Nothing enlivens a workout session like some good tunes. Creating a lively playlist with your loved one's favorite tracks can set the rhythm for exercise. Dancing to the beats, whether structured or freestyle, is not only a fantastic workout but also a mood enhancer. As a caregiver, occasionally shaking a leg with your loved one can foster deeper connections.
- Learning New Skills: Exercise doesn't always have to be traditional. How about signing up for a Tai Chi class or learning a new dance form? Such activities not only provide physical exercise but also stimulate the brain, making it a holistic experience. It's about movement, but it's also about growth, learning, and exploration.

As a caregiver, the key is approaching workouts with an open heart and mind. Your enthusiasm and participation can play a pivotal role in making exercise a joyous activity for your loved one. It's not about how intense the workouts are but how enjoyable they become.

MONITORING AND MEDICATIONS

Navigating the complex landscape of kidney disease is no simple task, especially when you're supporting a loved one through this journey. From understanding medications to employing modern technology for monitoring, a caregiver's role is multi-faceted. Let's delve deeper into how you can effectively support your loved one in managing their kidney health.

Administering Medicine

Medication plays a pivotal role in the management of kidney disease. It's instrumental in slowing down the progression of the illness, managing symptoms, and improving the overall quality of life for the patient. However, the effectiveness of these medicines hinges largely on their correct and consistent administration. As a caregiver, you are often the linchpin in this essential component of care. Here's a comprehensive guide to help you excel in this crucial role.

The Power of Punctuality: Most kidney medications work best when they are taken at consistent intervals. This consistency ensures that the therapeutic levels of the drug remain stable in the patient's system, maximizing efficacy. Set alarms or reminders to ensure that doses are not missed or delayed.

Reading and Understanding Prescriptions: It's crucial to thoroughly read and understand the dosing instructions. Does the medicine need to be taken with food, or should it be on an empty stomach? Are there any specific foods or drinks to avoid when on this medication? Such nuances can significantly impact the drug's effectiveness.

Organizing with Pill Organizers: A weekly or monthly pill organizer can be a game-changer, especially if multiple medicines are part of the regimen. Not only does it streamline the process, but it also provides a visual confirmation of whether the day's medications have been taken, reducing the risk of double dosing or missed doses.

Keeping Track: Maintain a medication journal or log. Note down any changes in symptoms, possible side effects, or any other observations. This can be invaluable information during doctor visits and can help in adjusting dosages or making medication changes if necessary.

Storing Medicines Correctly: Some medicines require specific storage conditions, like refrigeration or protection from light. Ensure that you're storing each medication as recommended to preserve its efficacy.

Staying Informed: It's beneficial to understand the purpose of each medicine. Is it to control blood pressure? Reduce proteinuria? Manage anemia? Knowing the 'why' behind each medication can provide clarity and purpose, making the regimen less daunting.

Preventing Drug Interactions: If the kidney patient is seeing multiple specialists, there's a possibility of drug interactions. Always keep an updated list of all medications, including over-the-counter ones, and share it with every healthcare provider. This ensures that any new prescription won't adversely interact with the current regimen.

Making It Palatable: Some medicines might have a distinct taste which can be off-putting. For oral medications, check with the pharmacist or doctor if it's okay to mix them with a small amount of food or drink to make them more palatable. However, be wary of grapefruit or grapefruit juice, as it can interact with many drugs.

Communication is Key: If the patient is experiencing difficulty with any medication, whether it's side effects, the mode of administration, or any other concern, communicate with the healthcare team. They can provide solutions, alternatives, or adjustments to the regimen.

Empathy and Patience: Remember, as a caregiver, your approach can set the tone. Administering medication might sometimes feel mechanical, but it's essential to remember the emotional aspects too. Encouraging words, a gentle touch, or just the act of listening can make the process smoother and more comfortable for your loved one.

While the science of medication is precise, the art of administering it requires a blend of organization, understanding, and empathy. By ensuring that medicines are taken correctly and consistently, you play a pivotal role in maximizing their benefits, helping to offer the kidney patient under your care the best chance at optimal health and quality of life.

Tracking Progress

For caregivers, managing a loved one's journey with kidney disease can feel like navigating a ship through stormy waters. As with any voyage, having accurate tools and measures to guide the way can make all the difference. Consistent tracking and monitoring of a kidney patient's health parameters can be likened to the compass and map on this journey. Let's unpack the depth of this essential practice, illustrating why it's pivotal and which metrics deserve meticulous attention.

The Essence of Continuous Observation: Kidney disease, with its ebbing and flowing nature, is a condition of complexities. Different periods can have contrasting characteristics - some may be tranquil with stable health parameters, while others might present unexpected challenges. This unpredictability underscores the need for an early detection system. Through systematic monitoring, even subtle shifts can be detected, allowing timely interventions and better-informed healthcare decisions.

Blood Pressure - The Pulse of Kidney Health: One cannot stress enough the intricate relationship between blood pressure and kidney health. Elevated blood pressure isn't just a risk factor for kidney disease but also a reflection of the ongoing kidney function. Monitoring blood pressure isn't just about numbers; it's about understanding the story those numbers tell. Acquiring a reliable home blood pressure monitor and noting readings consistently is imperative. Regular checks, preferably at the same time daily, can offer valuable insights into the effectiveness of medications and dietary practices.

Decoding Laboratory Narratives: Lab reports, while seemingly daunting with their medical jargon and numbers, are in reality the narrative of the kidney's state of affairs. Specific markers, such as serum creatinine, eGFR, and urine protein levels, provide a window into the kidneys' functional state. By methodically tracking these over intervals, caregivers can decipher patterns, thus enabling more targeted care strategies.

Physical Changes - The Silent Signals: Our bodies have an innate way of communicating, often silently. Whether it's the uncharacteristic swelling around the ankles, a subtle change in urine hue, or an unexplained fatigue, these are all the body's way of hinting at internal changes. A dedicated log, periodically updated, can be invaluable in tracking these signs.

Gauging Activity - A Reflection of Vitality: A person's activity level can often serve as a barometer for their overall well-being. Any drastic change, be it a surge in enthusiasm or an unexplained lethargy, can be indicative of underlying shifts in health. Employing tools like activity trackers can offer tangible data on this front.

Navigating Emotional Landscapes: The ripples of kidney disease extend beyond the physical realm, often casting shadows on emotional and mental well-being. Regular, open conversations and perhaps structured mental well-being checks can provide insights into a patient's psychological state. Emotional shifts might not just stem from the disease's progression but could also be side effects of medications.

Dietary Chronicles - The Vital Logs: Nutrition plays a colossal role in managing kidney disease. A meticulously kept food diary can be a goldmine of information. It serves a dual purpose - ensuring dietary guidelines are followed and helping establish links between specific foods and subsequent symptoms or wellness states.

The Pill Schedule - Ensuring Adherence: Medications, with their intricate timings and dosages, can be challenging to manage. Employing medication management tools, be they simple charts or digital platforms, can ensure adherence and help caregivers correlate any new symptoms with medication timings or changes.

Harnessing Digital Advancements: We live in a digital age, and healthcare isn't untouched by its blessings. From mobile applications that remind about medication timings to platforms that visualize health metrics trends, digital tools can simplify and enhance the tracking process.

Being a beacon of care in a kidney patient's journey necessitates an informed approach. Consistent, meticulous tracking is akin to the lighthouse guiding the ship, ensuring that the path taken is always aligned with the well-being and health of the loved one in focus.

Gadgets Galore: Embracing Technology

Home Blood Pressure Monitors: Having a reliable device at home provides the freedom to check blood pressure without clinical visits. Periodic calibration ensures its accuracy.

Oxygen Saturation Meters: For those showing respiratory

symptoms or those just curious, these devices provide real-time insights into oxygen levels in the bloodstream.

Advanced Scales: Modern scales do more than just weight. They offer data on hydration, bone density, and muscle mass. Such comprehensive metrics can inform dietary and exercise adjustments.

Medication Management Apps: With reminders, dosage information, and even interaction warnings, these apps are like having a mini-pharmacist in your pocket.

Nutrition Trackers: Aiding in dietary management, these apps can break down food intake into micro and macronutrients, essential for managing a renal diet. I, and most renal dietitians, recommend the app Cronometer. It has both a free version and a more advanced paid version. Let more about Cronometer at http://Go.DadviceTV.com/app

Activity Trackers: From steps taken to hours slept, modern fitness trackers provide a 360-degree view of one's activity levels. They can motivate and help set realistic health goals.

In the end, while technology can provide invaluable assistance, the human touch is irreplaceable. Use these tools to complement, not substitute, personal care and attention. These often go on sale or have manufacturer discounts, especially home blood pressure monitors. Check with your pharmacy to see what additional discounts or programs may be available.

When to Alert the Doctor

Being a caregiver to someone with kidney disease is a monumental responsibility. One of the essential tasks in this role is the vigilant observation of symptoms and understanding when to sound the alarm. Kidney disease, especially as it progresses, can manifest in a myriad of ways. These manifestations range from subtle signs to urgent, life-threatening symptoms. Recognizing them and responding promptly can mean the difference between routine treatment and a medical emergency.

The Weight Watch: Consistent monitoring of weight is crucial. A sudden increase might indicate fluid retention, a common issue with kidney dysfunction. Conversely, a swift decrease could suggest fluid loss or another underlying problem. Regular weight checks, preferably at the same time each day using the same scale, can offer invaluable data. Any variation exceeding 2-3 pounds in a day or 5 pounds in a week should be reported.

Swelling Spotting: Edema or swelling, especially in the ankles, hands, or face, is a tell-tale sign of fluid imbalance. While mild swelling after a long day can be common, persistent or severe swelling, especially if accompanied by other symptoms, requires attention.

Breathlessness: Shortness of breath might indicate two potential kidney-related issues: fluid buildup in the lungs or anemia. If someone experiences unexpected or severe breathlessness, especially if accompanied by chest pain or altered consciousness, it's time to call 911.

Tackling Fatigue: Constant fatigue or an unusual drop in energy levels can be a side effect of kidney disease. This could be due to anemia or toxin accumulation in the body. Regular blood tests can help monitor this, but any dramatic change in energy levels should be flagged.

Urine Urgency: Changes in urination patterns offer direct insights into kidney function. Whether it's an increase or decrease in frequency, noticeable differences in color, or the presence of blood, these changes are critical. Foamy or bubbly urine, in particular, can suggest protein loss and should be addressed.

Nausea Nuances: Feeling persistently nauseated or episodes of vomiting might suggest that the kidneys aren't efficiently filtering toxins. If over-the-counter remedies don't offer relief or if the issue is recurring, it's time to consult the nephrologist.

Taste and Breath Battles: A metallic taste in the mouth or a noticeable change in breath odor (often described as "ammonia breath") indicates toxin buildup. Regular oral hygiene can help, but persistent changes necessitate a doctor's visit.

Cold Comforts: Feeling cold consistently, particularly in the extremities, could be due to anemia or poor circulation related to kidney issues. While everyone feels cold now and then, if someone is wrapping up in blankets in warm weather, it's a sign.

Focus and Sleep Slips: Cognitive challenges, like concentration difficulties or disrupted sleep patterns, can be linked to mineral imbalances or toxin accumulation. Continuous monitoring and ensuring a stable sleep environment can help, but sudden or severe changes should be reported.

Skin Signals: Persistent itching, especially if accompanied by dryness, suggests mineral imbalance. While moisturizers can offer temporary relief, continuous discomfort, especially if it affects sleep, should be addressed with the healthcare team.

Lastly, always be prepared for emergencies. If any symptom feels severe, sudden, or if multiple symptoms present simultaneously, it might be time for emergency intervention. Symptoms like severe chest pain, dramatically altered consciousness, or intense difficulty breathing are immediate red flags. In such cases, always prioritize safety and call 911.

Being proactive, staying informed, and maintaining open lines of communication with the healthcare team ensures the best possible care and quality of life for the loved one under your care.

DOCTOR VISITS AND HOSPITAL STAYS

For individuals with kidney disease, frequent doctor visits and potential hospital stays become an integral part of their healthcare journey. These interactions with the medical world can be a lifeline, providing crucial monitoring, timely interventions, and essential guidance. For caregivers, understanding the intricacies of these appointments, recognizing what to expect, and ensuring a seamless experience for their loved ones is paramount. This chapter delves into the dynamics of doctor visits, hospital stays, and the associated preparations and considerations. It offers caregivers insights, resources, and strategies to navigate these experiences effectively, ensuring their loved ones receive the best possible care at every step.

Being the Advocate: A Pillar of Support and Clarity

The Power of Presence:
Being diagnosed with kidney disease is, for many, an overwhelming experience. Each doctor's appointment can feel like stepping into an alien world, fraught with medical jargon, complicated explanations, and a whirlwind of emotions. As a caregiver, your presence at these appointments serves as a beacon of familiarity and support. It's not just about being there physically; it's about being an active participant, helping to bridge the communication gap between the medical world and your loved one's reality.

Setting Appointments - The Groundwork:

The journey starts with setting the appointment. While it may seem straightforward, ensuring the preferred time slots, coordinating with work or other commitments, and accommodating for travel or recuperation times post-appointment is vital. Utilize digital platforms or traditional diaries to chalk out a calendar and align it with the patient's comfort and the doctor's availability.

Tracking Appointments - A Stitch in Time:
In the midst of caregiving responsibilities, it's easy to lose track of upcoming appointments. Employ reminders, be it through alarms, phone notifications, or even sticky notes on the refrigerator. Regularly reviewing the upcoming week's commitments can help in preemptively managing any clashes or rescheduling needs.

The Pre-Appointment Checklist:
Before the actual appointment, it's advantageous to prepare. Consider it akin to a strategic meeting. Gather recent lab reports, jot down any new symptoms or changes, and list down any questions or concerns. This not only ensures that pertinent issues are addressed but also maximizes the utility of the limited time with the doctor.

Punctuality - A Testament to Commitment:
Being punctual for appointments isn't just about respect for the doctor's time. It also ensures you have ample moments to settle down, organize thoughts, and even engage in preliminary discussions with nursing staff or assistants. Arriving a tad earlier can also help in administrative tasks, be it paperwork or insurance verifications.

Active Listening - The Art of Absorption:
Doctor's appointments, especially initial ones or those after significant tests, can be information-dense. As a caregiver, practice active listening. It's not just about hearing words but understanding the essence, asking for clarifications, and ensuring both you and the patient comprehend the medical

advice or directions provided.

Note-Taking - Archiving Medical Narratives:
Consider carrying a dedicated notebook or digital device for note-taking. Jotting down specifics, be it medication changes, recommended tests, or dietary suggestions, can be invaluable. These notes serve as a reference point and can be particularly useful for cross-referencing with past appointments or for future medical consultations.

The Power of Questions - Seeking Clarity:
Never hesitate to ask questions. If something is unclear, if a particular term seems alien, or if you're unsure about a specific instruction, seek clarity. Sometimes, the most crucial information surfaces when you probe or ask for elaborations.

Post-Appointment Reflections:
After the appointment, take a moment to review and reflect. Go over your notes, ensure the patient's understanding aligns with yours, and discuss any immediate actions or changes needed. This post-appointment review can often help in assimilating information and making it actionable.

Collaboration - The Heart of Healthcare:
Remember, healthcare, especially in chronic conditions like kidney disease, is collaborative. The doctor provides expertise, the patient shares their experiences, and you, the caregiver, act as the linchpin, bringing it all together. By being proactive, organized, and engaged, you're not just attending an appointment; you're actively championing your loved one's health journey.

In essence, as a caregiver during doctor visits, you play a multifaceted role. You're the advocate, the scribe, the clarifier, the supporter, and the organizer. By embracing each of these roles wholeheartedly, you ensure that every doctor's visit becomes a step forward in the journey towards better kidney health.

Hospital Bag Essentials

When supporting a loved one with kidney disease, one of the practical ways to be prepared is by packing an efficient hospital bag. Whether it's for regular doctor's appointments or an unexpected hospital stay, having a well-thought-out bag can make all the difference. Here's a detailed breakdown to ensure both comfort and utility.

Essentials for Doctor Visits:

Routine check-ups or specialist appointments can sometimes extend or lead to unplanned events. Being equipped can simplify the process.

- Complete Medication List: Bring along all current medications. This acts as an exact reference for the medical team. Include dosages, frequency, and the prescribing doctor's name, ensuring clarity. A printed list is handy for quick reviews.
- Medical Organizer: Apart from note-taking tools, keep a dedicated section for recent lab results, medical imaging, or any other pertinent documents. Keeping a digital copy on a thumb drive might also be useful.
- Insurance and ID: Always have an up-to-date insurance card and a photo ID. For ease, keep these in a dedicated pouch or section of the bag.
- Emergency Contact Sheet: While you, as a caregiver, are present, having an accessible list of other emergency contacts can be reassuring.

For Extended Hospital Stays:

An unplanned or even planned hospital admission requires some specific essentials. This list aims to merge the need for medical necessities with the comfort of home.

- Tech Essentials: A tablet or laptop, apart from

entertainment, can aid in research, communication, or even recording doctor instructions. Ensure these are password protected for security.
- Chargers and Power Banks: A multi-USB charger can power multiple devices. Power banks can be lifesavers during lengthy waits away from power outlets.
- Comfortable Clothing: Soft, easy-to-wear clothes like loungewear or pajamas can offer the comfort of home. Ensure they're front-opening if medical checks will be frequent. Slip-on shoes or non-slip socks can also be included.
- Personal Hygiene Kit: Create a compact hygiene kit with a toothbrush, toothpaste, unscented moisturizer, lip balm, face wash, a comb, and wet wipes. It's also beneficial to pack a quick-dry towel and a washcloth.
- Reading and Entertainment: Books, e-readers, magazines, or even audiobooks can help pass the time. Remember headphones if opting for digital entertainment.
- Eyecare: Along with glasses, if contact lenses are worn, include lens solution and a case. An eye mask can be handy for undisturbed sleep.
- Snack Pouch: Low-sodium, kidney-friendly snacks or nutrition bars can offer a familiar taste. Ensure to check dietary guidelines based on the current medical situation.
- Medication Overview: A detailed list of medications, timings, any allergies, and the respective prescribing doctor can facilitate accurate medical discussions.
- Leisure Activities: Crossword puzzles, coloring books, or portable board games can be engaging and act as stress relievers.
- Sleep Essentials: Hospitals can be bustling at all times.

Earplugs and an eye mask can help in creating a restful environment.
- Personal Touch: A comforting item, be it a cherished photograph, a favorite blanket, or a handwritten note, can uplift spirits and offer solace.
- Folder or Organizer: Keep a dedicated folder or organizer to collect and store any new documents, prescriptions, or information leaflets provided during the stay.

Being a caregiver requires both empathy and practicality. This comprehensive bag not only provides for the tangible needs but also communicates foresight, love, and care, ensuring the patient feels understood and supported.

Deciphering Lab Reports: A Comprehensive Guide for Caregivers

Kidney disease management hinges significantly on understanding laboratory tests, which are like a compass guiding the course of treatment. For caregivers, demystifying these lab reports is not just about interpreting numbers but understanding the narrative they weave about the patient's health. This narrative helps in taking proactive steps towards optimal kidney health and overall well-being.

A Closer Look at Kidney-Related Tests:
Delving into the details, let's discuss the various lab tests and their significance.

eGFR (Estimated Glomerular Filtration Rate)
- What it measures: eGFR is the cornerstone of kidney function assessment. It's derived from creatinine levels, age, body size, and gender.
- Understanding results: A reading between 90 to 120 is considered healthy. Values below 60 for a duration of three months or more suggest chronic kidney

disease.
- Management tips: A declining eGFR necessitates monitoring of blood pressure, blood sugar, adherence to a tailored renal diet, and potentially, medication adjustments.

Creatinine and Blood Urea Nitrogen (BUN)

- What they measure: These compounds result from metabolic processes - creatinine from muscle metabolism and BUN from protein metabolism.
- Understanding results: Elevated levels could mean the kidneys are struggling to filter out these wastes effectively.
- Management tips: Be vigilant about medication intake, and ensure dietary protein is consumed in appropriate amounts, tailored to the individual's kidney health.

Urinalysis and Proteinuria

- What it measures: Detects protein leakage in the urine.
- Understanding results: Kidneys should retain proteins; their presence in urine often flags kidney concerns.
- Management tips: Keep an eye on blood pressure and maintain open communication with the renal dietitian to adjust protein consumption if needed.

Potassium, Calcium, and Phosphorus Levels

- What they measure: These minerals and electrolytes play multifaceted roles in our bodies.
- Understanding results: Fluctuations in these levels can signal concerns related to muscle function, cardiac health, and bones.
- Management tips: Dietary changes often help

regulate these levels. For instance, elevated phosphorus might necessitate reducing phosphorus additives in foods.

Hemoglobin and Red Blood Cell Count

- What they measure: Hemoglobin is present in red blood cells and aids in transporting oxygen. The red blood cell count indicates the number of these oxygen-carrying cells.
- Understanding results: A dip in these levels often signifies anemia, a common ailment in CKD patients.
- Management tips: Consuming iron-rich foods or taking prescribed supplements can help. Erythropoiesis-stimulating agents might be needed in more severe cases.

PTH (Parathyroid Hormone)

- What it measures: It oversees the harmony between calcium and phosphorus in our body.
- Understanding results: Elevated PTH can suggest an imbalance in calcium and phosphorus, frequently observed in CKD.
- Management tips: Based on the results, calcium or vitamin D supplements might be prescribed.

A1C and Blood Sugar

- What they measure: A1C provides an average of blood sugar levels over the past three months, while blood sugar offers a snapshot of the current glucose level.
- Understanding results: Consistently high readings can indicate diabetes, a major risk factor and potential cause of kidney disease.
- Management tips: Managing carbohydrate intake,

taking prescribed medications, and regular exercise can help regulate these levels.

Sodium

- What it measures: Sodium levels in the bloodstream.
- Understanding results: Sodium imbalances can affect fluid balance and blood pressure.
- Management tips: Monitoring salt intake, especially from processed foods, is essential.

Iron Levels

- What they measure: Iron is crucial for hemoglobin production.
- Understanding results: Low iron can contribute to anemia.
- Management tips: Dietary sources like lean meats, beans, and iron-fortified foods can help. Supplements might be recommended based on the deficiency extent.

Vitamin D

- What it measures: Levels of this essential vitamin which aids in calcium absorption and bone health.
- Understanding results: Low levels can contribute to bone diseases.
- Management tips: Sun exposure, fortified foods, and supplements can be beneficial.

Uric Acid

- What it measures: Waste product from the metabolism of food.
- Understanding results: Elevated levels can lead to gout and are associated with kidney problems.
- Management tips: Avoiding high-purine foods like seafood and red meats, and staying hydrated can

help in managing uric acid levels.

Lab Reports: More Than Just Numbers:
For a caregiver, these reports are invaluable, telling stories of the kidney patient's health journey. They reveal patterns, guide interventions, and inform decisions. When reading a report, always remember:

- Document Everything: Maintaining an organized file or digital folder for all lab reports aids in drawing comparisons and noting patterns.
- Stay Engaged: Actively participate in medical visits. Take notes, seek clarifications, and ensure all concerns are addressed.
- Stay Updated and Research: Medical findings and guidelines evolve. Regularly update your knowledge about what each metric signifies and how it relates to the overall health of your loved one.
- Focus on the Trends: It's easy to get worried over a single value on a lab report, but it is normal for values to fluctuate. Stay focused on the trend, especially with the eGFR. Lab results are snapshots in time, and an eGFR may be slightly down from slight dehydration, and then back up the next time. The trend will show if the eGFR is stable or changing with time.

Lab tests and their reports are the bedrock of kidney disease management. By understanding their nuances, caregivers can offer more precise and holistic support to their loved ones, ensuring better health outcomes and improved quality of life.

Post-Visit Actions: Maximizing the Benefits of a Doctor's Appointment

After navigating the intricate dance of a doctor's appointment, the hours and days that follow are crucial. As a caregiver, your role does not end when the consultation door closes behind you.

Instead, it shifts towards ensuring the patient's adherence to the recommendations, understanding the nuances of the medical advice, and planning for subsequent steps. Here's how to ensure post-visit actions are as fruitful as the appointment itself:

Digesting the Information:

- After the visit, take a moment to reflect on the information shared. Doctor's appointments can be overwhelming, especially with a deluge of medical jargon. It's essential to process the advice, suggestions, and directives calmly and comprehensively.
- Don't hesitate to jot down any additional questions or concerns that arise after processing the information.

Reviewing and Organizing Prescriptions:

- If new medications were prescribed or changes were made to existing ones, it's vital to understand them. This includes dosage, frequency, and potential side effects.
- Organize medications in pill organizers, ensuring that they are stored correctly. Some might require refrigeration or protection from light.

Scheduling Follow-up Appointments:

- Doctors often suggest a follow-up to monitor progress or to assess how a new treatment is affecting the patient.
- Make sure you schedule these promptly to secure convenient dates and times. Input them in digital calendars or maintain a physical diary, setting reminders to ensure they aren't missed.

Research and Additional Learning:

- Sometimes, new terms, treatments, or diseases might have been discussed during the visit. Take the initiative

to research and understand these further. Trusted medical websites, kidney health forums, or academic publications can offer deeper insights.
- Stay cautious about the reliability of online sources. Always corroborate information from multiple trustworthy places.

Implement Dietary or Lifestyle Changes:
- If the doctor recommended specific lifestyle or dietary changes, begin incorporating them gradually into the daily routine. This can include new dietary guidelines, exercise routines, or stress-relieving activities.
- Consider consulting with specialists like renal dietitians or physical therapists for more targeted advice.

Communicate with Family:
- Share the outcomes of the visit with other family members. This ensures everyone is on the same page regarding the patient's health, any changes in treatment, or new observations.
- If there are complex procedures or treatments on the horizon, family discussions can provide collective insights and emotional support.

Maintain a Health Journal:
- Regularly update the patient's health journal. Log symptoms, moods, medication effects, or any other observations.
- This journal becomes a valuable resource during subsequent appointments, providing a comprehensive view of the patient's well-being.

Check for Test Results:
- If tests were conducted during the appointment, or if

the doctor ordered certain lab tests, keep track of when and how you'll receive these results.
- Don't hesitate to call the clinic or hospital if there are delays in receiving them.

Stay Financially Prepared:

- Understand the financial aspects of the visit, including billing, insurance claims, or out-of-pocket expenses. Address any discrepancies immediately.
- If new treatments or medications are suggested, review their cost implications and check if they are covered by insurance.

Open Channel with the Healthcare Team:

- Ensure that you have a clear line of communication with the doctor or the medical team for any questions or concerns that might arise post-visit.
- Many healthcare setups offer telehealth or online consultation facilities. Familiarize yourself with these, as they can be handy for quick clarifications.

By diligently following through with post-visit actions, caregivers play an instrumental role in bridging the gap between medical advice and its practical implementation. It's a continuum of care, ensuring that every doctor's visit translates into improved health and well-being for the kidney patient.

FINANCIAL AND LEGAL ASPECTS

Navigating the complexities of kidney disease is not just a medical journey but also a financial and legal expedition. As caregivers and loved ones of those diagnosed, understanding the intricacies of monetary and legal considerations becomes paramount. These aspects, often overshadowed by the immediate health concerns, play a pivotal role in ensuring long-term care, preserving quality of life, and safeguarding the patient's wishes and rights. This section delves into the crucial financial and legal dimensions associated with kidney disease, offering guidance, resources, and insights. It's vital to note that while this section provides a foundational understanding, everyone should consult with a family lawyer and financial advisor before taking any definitive action to ensure personalized, comprehensive planning.

Advanced Directive

Navigating the intricacies of kidney disease can be a daunting journey for patients and their caregivers. With various medical decisions and choices to be made along the way, it's imperative to have clarity on the patient's preferences, especially in situations where they might not be able to communicate those desires themselves. Enter the Advanced Directive, an essential tool that can provide peace of mind, clarity, and guidance during challenging times.

Understanding Advanced Directives

An Advanced Directive is a legal document that allows an individual to outline their decisions about end-of-life care ahead of time. It is a blueprint that guides family members and medical professionals on how to act if the person is unable to speak for themselves due to illness or incapacity.

Components of an Advanced Directive:
Typically, an Advanced Directive encompasses two main elements:

- Living Will: This is a written, legal document that spells out the types of medical treatments and life-sustaining measures you want—or don't want—such as mechanical breathing, tube feeding, or resuscitation.
- Durable Power of Attorney for Health Care: This element designates a person, often termed a health care proxy or agent, to make medical decisions on your behalf if you're unable to do so.

Legality and Variability:
Advanced Directives are legally valid throughout the United States, but laws and regulations vary from one state to another. It's crucial to be aware of your specific state's requirements and procedures.

The Importance for Kidney Patients

Kidney disease can be unpredictable. As it progresses, especially in advanced stages, patients might face significant health challenges that could render them unable to make or communicate decisions regarding their care.

Clarity in Crisis:
In emergencies, when quick decisions might be required, having an Advanced Directive in place ensures that the patient's wishes are known and can be followed. This clarity can be particularly crucial for kidney patients who may have specific concerns about treatments like dialysis or transplantation.

Reducing Emotional Strain:
Without an Advanced Directive, family members are left to guess what their loved one might want, which can lead to stress, uncertainty, and potential family disagreements. By clearly outlining their preferences, the patient provides a roadmap, reducing the emotional burden on the caregiver and other family members.

Personalization of Care:
Kidney patients often have unique and specific needs. An Advanced Directive allows them to lay down specific instructions tailored to their condition, ensuring care that aligns with their personal, cultural, or religious beliefs.

Role of the Caregiver

As a caregiver, your role in the process of creating an Advanced Directive is pivotal. You're not just a passive observer; you're an active participant, providing support, gathering information, and sometimes facilitating tough but necessary conversations.

Initiate the Dialogue:
Start the conversation with your loved one about the importance of drafting an Advanced Directive. Approach the topic with sensitivity, understanding, and patience.

Educate and Inform:
Equip yourself with knowledge. Understand what an Advanced Directive encompasses, the legalities involved, and the specifics as they pertain to kidney disease. Your knowledge can serve as a guiding light for your loved one as they navigate the process.

Facilitation:
Be there during the drafting process. Attend meetings with legal professionals, help gather necessary documents, and provide emotional support when discussing potentially challenging topics.

Review and Revisit:
An Advanced Directive isn't a one-time document. As the

patient's health condition evolves or if their wishes change, the directive may need updates. Regularly review the document and discuss any potential changes with your loved one.

In the complex journey of kidney disease, an Advanced Directive acts as a beacon, ensuring that the patient's wishes are respected and upheld. As a caregiver, your role in this process is invaluable. By championing the creation and maintenance of this crucial document, you're helping ensure that the journey, regardless of its twists and turns, remains patient-centered and in line with their desires and values.

Crafting an Advanced Directive

For caregivers assisting their loved ones in creating an Advanced Directive, understanding the sequential steps can provide a clear pathway. Let's delve into the systematic process of drafting an Advanced Directive:

1. Research and Familiarization

State-Specific Regulations: Begin by familiarizing yourself with the laws and regulations specific to the state or jurisdiction where the patient resides. Each state may have different forms, requirements, or terminologies associated with Advanced Directives.

2. Reflect on Health Care Wishes

Personal Choices: Encourage your loved one to think deeply about what they value most in terms of medical treatment. This includes decisions on resuscitation, life-support measures, pain management, organ donation, and more.

3. Engage in Conversations

Open Dialogues: Talk with family members, close friends, religious leaders, and, importantly, health care providers about the patient's wishes. These conversations ensure that everyone understands and respects the decisions made.

4. Choose a Health Care Proxy

Selecting an Agent: An essential part of the Advanced Directive is appointing a health care proxy or agent. This person will make decisions on the patient's behalf if they're incapacitated. The chosen individual should be trustworthy, understanding of the patient's wishes, and capable of making potentially challenging decisions under pressure.

5. Documentation

Utilize Forms: Most states provide standardized Advanced Directive forms. These can be obtained from health departments, senior centers, your physician's office, or online.

Specify Instructions: Ensure that the document clearly outlines the patient's medical preferences, including details about specific treatments and interventions they desire or want to avoid.

6. Seek Legal Counsel (If Necessary)

While not always required, in some states or complex situations, consulting with an attorney who specializes in health care directives might be beneficial.

7. Witnessing and Notarization

Some states require Advanced Directives to be witnessed or notarized. Ensure that you follow your state's specific guidelines about who can act as a witness.

8. Distribute Copies

Once the Advanced Directive is finalized, make multiple copies. Distribute them to the health care proxy, family members, primary care physicians, specialists, and hospitals where the patient might be treated. Keeping a digital copy can also be handy.

9. Regular Reviews

Update as Necessary: Health wishes and life situations can evolve. Encourage periodic reviews of the Advanced Directive, especially after significant life events or changes in health status.

10. Communicate Changes

If any changes are made to the Advanced Directive, be sure to communicate these to all parties involved. This ensures everyone is up-to-date with the latest decisions and wishes.

Drafting an Advanced Directive is a profound act of autonomy and love. By outlining clear health care decisions in advance, it alleviates the burden on family and ensures that, even in critical moments, the patient's voice is heard and respected. As a caregiver, guiding your loved one through this process is an invaluable service, one that provides clarity and peace in challenging times.

Power of Attorney

When navigating the complexities of health challenges like kidney disease, it's paramount to understand and implement legal tools that can assist in decision-making. One such tool is the Power of Attorney (POA). Let's delve into what it means and how it can be set up, especially in the context of kidney disease.

1. Definition of Power of Attorney

A Power of Attorney is a legal document that allows an individual (known as the "principal") to grant another person (the "agent" or "attorney-in-fact") the authority to make decisions on their behalf. This can cover a range of matters, including financial, medical, or other personal affairs.

2. Types of Power of Attorney

- General Power of Attorney: Grants broad powers to an agent to act on behalf of the principal in various matters such as financial transactions or business dealings.
- Durable Power of Attorney: Remains in effect even if the principal becomes mentally incapacitated. This is crucial for individuals with medical conditions that

might impact their cognitive abilities.
- Medical Power of Attorney: Specifically allows the agent to make health care decisions for the principal if they are unable to do so. This can be invaluable for individuals with advanced kidney disease, especially if they reach a stage where they can't communicate their health care wishes.

3. Importance for Kidney Disease Patients

For those diagnosed with kidney disease, health can be unpredictable. As the disease progresses, patients might face situations where they are unable to make decisions for themselves due to physical or mental incapacitation. Having a designated POA—particularly a Medical Power of Attorney—ensures that someone trusted can step in and make decisions in line with the patient's desires.

4. Steps to Designate a Power of Attorney

- Evaluate Needs: Determine the type of POA required based on current health and future concerns. For kidney disease patients, considering a Medical Power of Attorney alongside a general or durable one might be beneficial.
- Choose a Trusted Agent: Select someone reliable, understanding, and capable of making decisions in alignment with the principal's wishes. This could be a family member, close friend, or even a legal professional.
- Consult an Attorney: While there are many standardized POA forms available, consulting with an attorney ensures that the document adheres to state-specific regulations and truly captures the principal's wishes.
- Clearly Define Powers: Be specific about the authority being granted. This ensures the agent understands

their responsibilities and limits.
- Sign and Notarize: Most states require the POA to be signed in the presence of witnesses, and some might need the document to be notarized.
- Distribute Copies: Provide copies to the designated agent, health care providers, financial institutions, and other relevant parties. This ensures that, when the time comes, there are no delays in executing the POA.

5. Periodic Review

Life circumstances and health statuses change. Review the POA periodically, especially after major life events or significant shifts in health. If amendments are needed, it's much like the initial setup process: make the changes, sign, notarize, and distribute updated copies.

6. Revocation of Power of Attorney

If the principal decides to change their agent or revoke the powers given, they can do so as long as they are mentally competent. The revocation should be in writing, and all concerned parties should be informed.

Financial Planning

Caring for a loved one with kidney disease involves more than understanding medical needs. It's also about navigating the financial labyrinth associated with chronic illnesses. As treatment costs can pile up quickly, having a sound financial strategy in place is paramount. Let's delve into the intricate facets of financial planning for kidney disease and provide caregivers with tools to manage expenses.

Grasping the Full Picture of Kidney Disease Costs

Understanding Medical Treatments: Kidney disease brings along a series of medical procedures that vary in cost. From initial consultations to medications, dialysis sessions, and potentially, transplant surgeries – it's crucial to be aware of these expenses.

Hidden Costs: Beyond the obvious medical bills, consider costs like transportation to medical appointments, dietary needs, home modifications for dialysis, and even over-the-counter supplements or vitamins.

Long-Term Implications: It's essential to recognize that kidney disease is a long-term condition. This isn't just about managing immediate costs but preparing for expenses that could span decades.

Crafting a Financial Roadmap

Setting Clear Budgets: Establish a comprehensive budget. Factor in all regular expenses, then allocate a segment for expected medical costs.

Emergency Reserves: Always anticipate unforeseen costs. Establishing a dedicated emergency fund can mitigate financial shocks from unexpected treatments or complications.

Financial Counseling: A professional, especially one with experience in medical costs, can guide you in budgeting, insurance considerations, and potential financial aid sources.

Navigating the Insurance Maze

Health Insurance: Comprehensive health insurance is invaluable. Examine your current policy to ensure it covers kidney-related treatments. If shopping for new insurance, prioritize those that cover chronic disease treatments extensively.

Medicare and Medicaid: Beyond regular insurance, those with kidney disease might qualify for Medicare or Medicaid. These government programs can drastically reduce out-of-pocket costs. Remember, each state might have slightly different Medicaid rules, so familiarize yourself with your state's criteria.

Additional Coverage: Supplemental insurance policies can cover gaps in traditional insurance. These can be instrumental in managing co-pays or treatments not fully covered by primary insurance.

Dialysis, Medications, and More: Managing Core Expenses

Pharmaceutical Aid: Some drug manufacturers offer assistance programs, granting patients access to medications at reduced prices or sometimes even for free. Always inquire about such programs when prescribed a new medication.

Treatment Center Financial Programs: Many dialysis centers or hospitals provide financial assistance or flexible payment structures. Discussing your financial concerns with them can open doors to cost-saving measures you weren't aware of.

Preparing for Potential Transplants

Transplant surgeries, while life-saving, come with a significant price tag. However, several non-profits, such as the National Foundation for Transplants or the American Transplant Foundation, can assist with these costs. Moreover, consider the post-surgery costs, like anti-rejection medications, which are a lifelong expense.

Always Keep Track

Routine Check on Bills: Medical billing errors can happen. Regularly checking and questioning discrepancies can save substantial amounts over time.

Financial Health Checks: Just as your loved one will have regular medical checkups, periodically review your financial strategy. Adjust budgets as necessary, keeping an eye out for areas where you might save.

Fostering Open Communication with Healthcare Providers

Your loved one's healthcare team is an invaluable resource, not just medically but financially as well. They can suggest alternative treatments, medications, or procedures that are more cost-effective. Establish a rapport, ask questions, and never hesitate to discuss financial concerns.

Safeguarding the Future

Given the long-term nature of kidney disease, consider investments like long-term care insurance. It can be beneficial if full-time care becomes necessary. Disability insurance can also be a saving grace if the patient's ability to work becomes compromised.

Staying Informed Equals Financial Preparedness

Healthcare laws, policies, and even treatment costs change. Being proactive by staying informed can position you to make the best financial decisions for your loved one's care.

In this journey with kidney disease, while ensuring the best medical care is pivotal, it's equally essential to shield your family from potential financial strains. With adequate planning, diligence, and a proactive approach, you can effectively manage the financial challenges that come with kidney disease.

Fundraising and Support: Navigating Financial Relief

In the world we live in today, the costs associated with chronic illnesses like kidney disease can quickly become overwhelming. While health insurance and personal savings play a pivotal role in addressing these expenses, there are moments when they might not suffice. Here's where the power of community, both offline and online, can make a considerable difference.

Tapping into Community Strength: Our communities, be it our neighborhood, church, workplace, or broader social circles, often rally around those in need. Organizing local fundraisers, such as bake sales, car washes, or charity auctions, can garner both monetary support and heightened awareness about kidney disease.

Digital Crowdfunding Platforms: Websites like GoFundMe have revolutionized the fundraising landscape. They offer a platform where individuals can share their stories and seek financial assistance. However, it's heartbreaking to acknowledge that such platforms have become almost essential for many to meet their healthcare costs. While they provide a lifeline, their necessity underscores a broader issue with the healthcare system's affordability.

Benefits of Online Fundraising: Digital platforms amplify reach. Your story can resonate with people globally, and donations can pour in from unexpected quarters. Additionally, these platforms usually offer secure payment gateways, ensuring the money raised reaches you safely.

Harnessing Social Media: Platforms like Facebook, Instagram, or Twitter can be instrumental in spreading the word about your fundraising campaign. Sharing regular updates about the patient's health journey can keep well-wishers informed and encourage more people to contribute.

Local Organizations and Non-profits: Several local bodies and non-profits assist families grappling with medical expenses. From providing funds to connecting families with potential donors, their support can be invaluable.

Employer Assistance: Some companies have programs to assist employees undergoing financial distress due to medical reasons. They might match donations, provide grants, or even offer paid time off.

Transparent Communication: While seeking funds, maintaining transparency about expenses, treatment plans, and progress can build trust. Donors often appreciate knowing how their contributions are making a difference.

Mental and Emotional Benefits: Beyond financial relief, fundraising campaigns often shower the affected family with emotional and moral support. Reading encouraging messages from donors, hearing stories from others who've been on similar journeys, or just knowing people care can be immensely uplifting.

Always Express Gratitude: A simple 'Thank You' goes a long way. Acknowledging contributors, no matter how small their donation, fosters goodwill and strengthens community bonds.

The financial strains associated with kidney disease can be daunting. But, with a combination of community support, digital platforms, and sheer determination, many families find a way to weather this storm. Embracing the strength of collective efforts not only aids in meeting costs but also instills hope and courage in the journey ahead.

LONG-TERM CARE AND DIALYSIS SUPPORT

The journey of managing kidney disease is multifaceted and can lead to various treatment avenues. One such pivotal treatment, which many have heard of but might not fully grasp, is dialysis. While the primary focus of this book has been on providing insights for kidney patients who are not on dialysis, it's paramount to understand the scope and intricacies of dialysis, especially for caregivers. This chapter intends to shed light on the fundamental aspects of dialysis, its types, and how it impacts daily life, all while underscoring the significant role caregivers play in this phase of kidney care.

What Is Dialysis?

Dialysis acts as an artificial kidney, a treatment designed to filter and purify the blood when the kidneys can no longer perform this function adequately. Its primary role is to remove excess waste, salt, and water, thereby maintaining a balance of various elements like potassium and sodium in the blood.

There are mainly two types of dialysis:

- Hemodialysis: The most common type, hemodialysis, involves circulating blood outside of the body through a machine that filters out the waste products. It's usually done in a specialized center three times a week, with each session lasting about three to five hours.

- Peritoneal Dialysis: This method involves the insertion of a catheter into the abdomen. A dialysate solution captures waste products as it washes in and out of the abdomen. There are different variations of peritoneal dialysis, but it's usually done daily at home.

The decision to start dialysis isn't made lightly. Current kidney guidelines often suggest initiating dialysis when eGFR (estimated glomerular filtration rate) drops between 5-7. However, there are instances when it might be started earlier due to uncontrollable symptoms or other associated risk factors.

Homecare Guidelines

Being on dialysis, especially if it's done at home, involves a significant adjustment to one's daily life. For caregivers, understanding the patient's needs post-dialysis is crucial to ensure their well-being.

- Post-Dialysis Fatigue: It's common for patients to feel drained or tired after a dialysis session. Having a comfortable resting space ready, with pillows and blankets, can be comforting.
- Dietary Needs: While dialysis clears many waste products from the blood, dietary modifications continue to be essential. Providing a balanced meal, keeping in mind any restrictions or changes recommended by their renal dietitian, is vital.
- Hydration: Although overhydration can be a concern for dialysis patients, they still need to drink fluids. Offering them a glass of water or herbal tea can be soothing, especially after hemodialysis.
- Medication: Ensure they take post-dialysis medications, if any, as prescribed. Keep a chart or a digital tracker to ensure consistency.
- Monitor for Complications: Watch out for any signs

of infection, especially if they're on peritoneal dialysis. This includes redness, swelling, or unusual discharge around the catheter site.
- Emotional Support: Dialysis can be emotionally taxing. Offering a listening ear, spending quality time, or even watching a movie together can provide much-needed comfort.
- Exercise: While it's essential to rest post-dialysis, encouraging light activities or exercises on non-dialysis days can be beneficial for their overall health.

For caregivers, being attentive to these needs and staying informed about potential changes in the patient's condition is of paramount importance. The support provided during this phase can make a significant difference in the patient's quality of life.

Choosing A Dialysis Center

Selecting the right dialysis center is a crucial decision for both the kidney patient and their caregivers. It's not merely about finding a facility; it's about selecting a center that aligns with the patient's medical, emotional, and logistical needs. Below are factors to consider when evaluating dialysis centers:

- Location: The proximity of the center to the patient's home is vital. Given the frequency of treatments, choosing a center close to home can reduce travel fatigue and expenses.
- Accreditation and Certification: Ensure that the center is accredited by relevant health bodies and meets all state and federal standards. A center's certification can give you an idea about the quality of care they provide.
- Medical Staff: The expertise and experience of the medical staff, including nephrologists, nurses, and technicians, play a significant role. It's beneficial to inquire about the training and qualifications of the

staff members.
- Patient-to-Staff Ratio: A lower patient-to-staff ratio often means more personalized care and attention during treatments.
- Types of Dialysis Offered: Some centers might offer both hemodialysis and peritoneal dialysis, while others might specialize in one. Depending on the patient's requirements, ensure that the chosen method is available.
- Availability of Support Services: Centers that offer support services such as dietary counseling, social work services, or psychological counseling can be advantageous for holistic care.
- Cleanliness and Hygiene: The overall cleanliness of the center is a paramount consideration, given the risk of infections. Regularly cleaned and well-maintained facilities indicate a higher standard of care.
- Emergency Protocols: It's essential to know how the center handles emergencies. Do they have the necessary equipment and trained staff to manage unexpected medical situations?
- Schedule Flexibility: Some centers might offer more flexible dialysis schedules, including evening or weekend slots, which can be more convenient for patients and their caregivers.
- Patient Reviews and Feedback: Talking to current or past patients can provide insights into the real-time experience at the center. Online reviews and ratings might also be helpful, though they should be taken with a grain of caution.
- Cost and Insurance: Understanding the cost structure and whether the center accepts your insurance is essential. Some centers might also offer financial

- counseling to help navigate insurance and payment options.
- Ambiance and Comfort: A comfortable and friendly environment can make the dialysis experience less daunting. Look for centers that prioritize patient comfort, from reclining chairs to entertainment options during treatment.
- Opportunities for Education: Centers that offer education sessions or workshops for patients and caregivers can be beneficial. These sessions can help in understanding the disease better and managing it more effectively.

While the technical and medical aspects of a dialysis center are undeniably crucial, the human touch, compassion, and understanding they offer can make a world of difference to the patient's overall experience. As caregivers, your active participation in this selection process can provide immense support to your loved one in their journey.

Dialysis At Home

Dialysis at home, as the name suggests, allows kidney patients to undergo dialysis treatments in the comfort of their own homes rather than visiting a dialysis center regularly. This method of treatment has been gaining traction and is becoming increasingly accessible for many due to its range of benefits. Let's delve into an overview of dialysis at home and its inherent advantages.

Understanding Dialysis at Home

There are two main types of dialysis treatments that can be conducted at home:

- Home Hemodialysis (HHD): This method uses a machine to clean the patient's blood, similar to the machines used at dialysis centers. However, the

machines designed for home use are typically smaller and more user-friendly. Regular training is provided to both patients and caregivers to ensure they can manage the equipment safely and efficiently.
- Peritoneal Dialysis (PD): Instead of using a machine to clean the blood, PD uses a special fluid infused into the patient's abdomen through a catheter. This fluid absorbs the waste from the blood through the peritoneal membrane in the abdomen. After a set period, the used fluid is drained and replaced with fresh fluid.

Benefits of Dialysis at Home

- Flexibility: One of the most significant advantages is the flexibility in scheduling. Patients aren't restricted to the fixed schedules of a dialysis center. This flexibility can significantly enhance the quality of life, allowing for a better balance of work, recreation, and treatment.
- Comfort and Familiarity: Undergoing treatment in a familiar environment can reduce the anxiety and stress associated with regular hospital visits. Patients can watch their favorite shows, read, or even sleep in their beds during the process.
- Reduced Travel: Eliminating the need for frequent trips to a dialysis center can save time, reduce travel expenses, and decrease the wear and tear of regular travel, especially beneficial for those who don't live near a treatment center.
- Personalized Care: With home dialysis, there's an opportunity for more frequent or extended sessions, which some studies suggest can offer better health outcomes. This flexibility allows treatments to be tailored more closely to the patient's needs.

- Increased Independence: For many, the ability to manage their treatment empowers them, giving them a sense of control over their disease.
- Potential for Better Health Outcomes: Some studies have indicated that more frequent home dialysis can lead to better blood pressure control, reduced dietary restrictions, and improved symptoms, such as fatigue or nausea.
- Cost-Efficiency: In some cases, home dialysis can be more cost-effective. This cost efficiency can be due to reduced transportation costs, fewer medications, and fewer hospitalizations.
- Supportive Environment: Being surrounded by loved ones can offer emotional and psychological support, making the treatment process more bearable and improving mental well-being.

While home dialysis offers multiple benefits, it's crucial to note that it might not be suitable for everyone. Consultation with healthcare professionals is essential to determine if it's the right choice for the patient. However, for those who are eligible and choose this route, home dialysis can be a game-changer, offering a combination of medical efficacy and improved quality of life.

THE PSYCHOLOGICAL ASPECTS OF CARING FOR SOMEONE WITH KIDNEY DISEASE

Taking care of someone with kidney disease is a journey, not only for the patient but also for the caregiver. Kidney disease brings with it a myriad of challenges, both physical and psychological. Understanding these challenges and being equipped to deal with them is vital for the overall well-being of both the patient and the caregiver. One significant aspect of this caregiving journey is addressing the psychological needs of the patient and understanding the emotional toll it might take on the caregiver. There is great importance in seeking professional guidance, especially from a therapist, in managing stress and ensuring that anxiety does not spiral out of control. This chapter will delve deep into the psychological realm of caregiving for kidney disease patients and offer insights and strategies to navigate this often-overlooked aspect of care.

Finding a Therapist

Locating Mental Health Resources:
Finding a suitable therapist is the first step towards addressing the emotional and psychological needs of a kidney disease

patient. Local health departments, hospitals, and clinics often maintain a list of licensed therapists in the community. Moreover, organizations like the National Kidney Foundation and the American Psychological Association offer directories and resources to help locate mental health professionals experienced in handling the challenges specific to kidney disease.

Benefits of Seeing a Therapist:
Therapists provide a safe space for patients and caregivers to express their feelings, fears, and frustrations. They can offer guidance on coping strategies, provide emotional support, and assist in addressing any psychological disorders that may arise, such as depression or anxiety. Engaging in therapy can lead to better emotional well-being, which can have a positive effect on the physical health of the kidney patient.

When to Seek a Therapist:
While it's never too early or too late to seek therapy, there are certain signs that indicate it might be particularly beneficial. If the patient or caregiver is feeling persistently sad, anxious, or overwhelmed; if there are strains in personal relationships; or if there's a general feeling of being unable to cope with the demands of the disease, it might be time to consider professional help.

Family Coping Strategies

Understanding the Emotional Impact:
Kidney disease is a life-altering diagnosis that affects the entire family unit. Emotions like shock, denial, anger, sadness, and anxiety can surface not only in the patient but also among family members. Recognizing and addressing these emotions is paramount in ensuring the well-being of everyone involved.

Managing Stress:
Undoubtedly, caregiving can lead to heightened stress levels. Here are some strategies to keep stress in check:

- Regular Breaks: Intermittently stepping away from caregiving duties, even if just for a short while, can help rejuvenate the mind and body.
- Support Groups: Joining support groups where one can share experiences, concerns, and solutions with others in similar situations can be therapeutic.
- Educate: Knowledge is empowering. Understanding kidney disease and its implications can lessen anxiety stemming from the unknown. Utilizing resources, such as books, websites, and seminars, can be instrumental.
- Delegate: Sharing responsibilities among family members can distribute the workload and reduce individual strain.

Communication is Key:
Keeping an open line of communication is essential to ensure that everyone's needs and concerns are addressed.

- Regular Family Meetings: Designate a time for the family to come together and discuss caregiving roles, challenges, and emotional well-being. This fosters understanding and collaboration.
- Seek Feedback: Encourage family members to voice their concerns, suggestions, or anything they feel might help in the caregiving process.
- Stay Informed: If possible, accompany the patient to medical appointments. This ensures that everyone has the latest information on the patient's condition and care requirements.

Establishing Boundaries:
For the caregiver's well-being, it's crucial to establish boundaries.

- Set Limits: Recognize that one cannot be available

for caregiving duties 24/7. Determine what you can reasonably do and communicate that to the patient and other family members.
- Prioritize Self-care: While it's easy to get caught up in caring for the patient, neglecting one's own health and well-being can lead to burnout. Set aside time for activities you love, whether it's reading, gardening, or simply taking a long bath.
- Professional Help: If the emotional toll becomes overwhelming, consider seeking professional counseling or therapy. It's essential for caregivers to recognize when they need assistance.

Engage in Activities as a Family:
Finding activities that the entire family can participate in can serve as a respite from the daily routine and strengthen familial bonds.

- Outdoor Activities: A simple picnic in the park, short hikes, or even a walk around the neighborhood can be refreshing.
- Board Games and Movie Nights: These are great ways to engage with family members in a relaxed setting.
- Cooking Together: Preparing meals together not only divides the task but also provides an opportunity for bonding. This can also be a chance to explore and experiment with kidney-friendly recipes.

Through understanding, collaboration, and effective communication, families can navigate the complexities of kidney disease with resilience and compassion, ensuring that both the patient and caregivers feel supported and understood.

Mindfulness Techniques

Understanding Mindfulness:

Mindfulness is a profound practice rooted in ancient traditions but has found significant relevance in today's fast-paced world. It revolves around the principle of being fully immersed in the present moment, observing thoughts and feelings without judgment. For caregivers of kidney disease patients, this can provide a sanctuary from the whirlwind of responsibilities and emotional burdens, enabling them to return to their roles rejuvenated and with a clear mind.

Deep Breathing:
Taking slow, deep breaths, in through the nose and out through the mouth, has a therapeutic effect on the mind and body. It shifts the body from a state of stress (sympathetic nervous system activation) to a state of relaxation (parasympathetic nervous system activation). Regular deep breathing sessions, even for just a few minutes daily, can be immensely beneficial.

Progressive Muscle Relaxation:
This method involves consciously tensing and then relaxing different muscle groups in the body. By focusing on the sensation of tension and release, caregivers can become more attuned to physical sensations and divert their attention away from overwhelming thoughts. Over time, this practice helps in reducing overall physical tension and fostering relaxation.

Guided Imagery:
This involves visualizing calming and serene environments or situations, such as a quiet beach, a tranquil forest, or floating on a cloud. The vividness of the imagery can have a profound calming effect, transporting the individual away from immediate stressors. Numerous apps and audio recordings offer guided imagery sessions tailored for relaxation and stress relief.

Meditation:
While there are various forms of meditation, the essence remains the same: focusing the mind and eliminating the stream of jumbled thoughts that may be crowding one's head. Starting with just a few minutes daily and gradually increasing

the duration can lead to enhanced mental clarity and reduced anxiety. Techniques such as loving-kindness meditation, body scan meditation, and breath awareness meditation can be particularly helpful for caregivers.

Mindful Walking:
Transforming regular walks into mindful walks can be revitalizing. This involves walking slowly and being fully aware of every step, feeling the ground beneath, noticing the rhythm of the breath, and being attuned to the surroundings. Such walks can be a form of moving meditation, offering both physical and mental benefits.

Journaling:
Writing down thoughts and feelings can be a form of mindfulness practice. It offers an opportunity to reflect, gain clarity, and process emotions. For caregivers, maintaining a regular journal can serve as both a therapeutic outlet and a record of their caregiving journey.

Yoga:
While yoga is often associated with physical postures, its essence is deeply rooted in mindfulness. The synchronicity of breath and movement in yoga not only enhances physical well-being but also promotes mental calmness and focus. Even simple poses or sequences, when done mindfully, can be restorative.

Embracing these mindfulness techniques can be a transformative experience for caregivers. Integrating them into daily routines can provide a much-needed anchor amidst the challenges, bringing moments of calm, clarity, and rejuvenation.

EMPLOYMENT WITH KIDNEY DISEASE

The diagnosis of kidney disease, while challenging, doesn't automatically mean an end to regular professional engagements for the patient. In fact, many individuals with kidney disease continue to lead fulfilling work lives, with some adjustments and considerations. Most kidney patients are able to continue their employment with minimal to no disruptions. However, for some, addressing physical challenges such as anemia-induced low energy, frequent medical appointments, or accommodating dialysis schedules may become imperative. Open communication with the employer, especially the Human Resources department, can pave the way for a more accommodating and kidney-friendly work environment. By understanding and addressing the unique needs of an employee with kidney disease, both the employee and employer can find ways to ensure productivity and well-being.

Workplace Challenges

While the determination and resilience of many kidney patients allow them to excel in their professional lives, there are undeniable challenges that they might face in the workplace. By understanding these challenges, both employers and colleagues can play a role in creating an environment that is supportive and accommodating.

Balancing Work and Medical Needs:
The intertwining of professional duties and medical necessities is a delicate dance.

- Medical Appointments: Regular check-ups, tests, and other appointments can sometimes consume a significant portion of the workweek. While some appointments can be scheduled outside of working hours, others might not offer such flexibility.
- Dialysis Schedules: For patients undergoing dialysis, the treatment sessions, which could be multiple times a week, may intersect with work hours. Some patients might opt for nocturnal dialysis to mitigate its impact on their workday, but this isn't always feasible for everyone.
- Energy Levels and Productivity: Kidney disease can sometimes lead to reduced energy levels, which can affect productivity. Moments of fatigue might not align with traditional break times, making it necessary to rest at unconventional hours.

Emotional and Mental Health Challenges:
The emotional weight of managing a chronic condition can sometimes be overwhelming.

- Anxiety and Stress: Concerns about health, potential medical complications, or maintaining job performance can lead to heightened levels of anxiety. Chronic stress can exacerbate kidney disease symptoms and further impact work performance.
- Cognitive Challenges: Some patients might experience cognitive changes due to their condition, affecting their memory, attention span, or ability to process information quickly.

Social and Interpersonal Challenges:

How kidney disease impacts social interactions in a professional setting is also worth noting.

- Perceptions and Misunderstandings: A lack of awareness about kidney disease can lead to misconceptions. Colleagues might misconstrue reduced energy levels as a lack of interest or commitment.
- Isolation: Due to dietary restrictions or the need to avoid potential infections, some kidney patients might refrain from participating in social events, office get-togethers, or group lunches, leading to feelings of isolation.

Physical Environment Challenges:
The typical office environment might present its own set of challenges.

- Accessibility: If the office is spread over multiple floors, ensuring easy accessibility to all essential areas, especially for those who might experience fatigue, is crucial.
- Restroom Access: Given the importance of hydration for kidney patients, easy and frequent access to restrooms becomes vital.
- Temperature Sensitivities: Some kidney patients might be more sensitive to cold. Ensuring a comfortable ambient temperature or providing space heaters can make a difference.

Addressing workplace challenges requires a collaborative effort. With open communication, understanding, and a few adjustments, kidney patients can continue to thrive professionally while managing their health effectively.

Work Environment Modifications

Creating a kidney-friendly work environment is not just about ensuring physical comfort; it's also about fostering a sense of inclusivity and understanding. A conducive workplace can significantly enhance the professional experience for kidney patients, making them feel valued and supported. Here are further modifications and considerations that can be beneficial:

Physical Workspace Adjustments:
The actual workspace should promote comfort, ease of movement, and overall well-being.

- Adjustable Workstations: Desks that can be adjusted for both sitting and standing can be particularly beneficial. This allows the employee to change their position based on comfort throughout the day.
- Supportive Footrests: Given that some kidney patients may retain fluid, having an adjustable footrest can help them elevate their feet, reducing swelling.
- Optimal Lighting: Proper lighting reduces eye strain. Adjustable lights, or even desk lamps, can be introduced so that employees can set lighting levels according to their preference.

Health and Wellness Facilities:
Facilities that cater to the overall well-being of the employee can be invaluable.

- Quiet Rooms: Designating a quiet room or space where employees can relax, meditate, or even nap can be beneficial, especially for those dealing with fatigue.
- Health Workshops: Organizing workshops on topics like stress management, nutrition, or general wellness can be beneficial for all employees, not just those with kidney disease.
- Physical Activity Encouragements: If possible, introducing light physical activity breaks, like stretch

sessions or short walks, can be beneficial. This not only aids physical health but also serves as a mental break.

Open Policy on Medical Equipment:
Some kidney patients might require medical equipment, even at work.

- Space for Medical Equipment: Ensure there's a provision for storage or use of any medical equipment, like a peritoneal dialysis machine, if the patient opts for mid-day sessions at work.
- Refrigeration Access: If medications need to be stored at a cool temperature, providing access to a refrigerator is essential.

Regular Feedback Mechanism:
To ensure that the modifications are effective and address the employee's needs, a feedback mechanism should be in place.

- Anonymous Surveys: Regularly conducting anonymous surveys can help employees voice their comfort level with the current modifications and suggest improvements.
- Dedicated HR Point of Contact: Having a dedicated person within Human Resources whom employees can approach with their concerns or needs ensures that they always have a channel for communication.

Education and Awareness Programs:
The more the workforce understands kidney disease, the more supportive the environment.

- Awareness Workshops: Organizing sessions where employees are educated about kidney disease, its implications, and how they can support their colleagues can foster a more understanding workplace.
- Informational Brochures: Distributing brochures or pamphlets that shed light on kidney disease can also

aid in raising awareness.

By taking a proactive approach and making thoughtful modifications, employers can create a work environment that acknowledges the unique challenges faced by kidney patients, ensuring they feel supported, valued, and empowered to perform to the best of their abilities.

FINDING COMMUNITY SUPPORT

Navigating the complexities of kidney disease is a journey that no one should walk alone. While the medical and physical challenges are apparent, the emotional and psychological burdens can be just as taxing. For caregivers, the responsibility often goes beyond ensuring the patient's well-being; they must also manage their own emotional health. Thankfully, one doesn't have to look far to find a community of individuals who understand, empathize, and offer support. From local groups to global online communities, there's a myriad of avenues to find the help, advice, and camaraderie that can make this journey a shared one. This chapter delves into the various sources of community support available to caregivers and patients alike, emphasizing the importance of connectivity and mutual understanding.

Local Support Groups

Local support groups play an indispensable role in providing hands-on, face-to-face interaction, which can be therapeutic and reassuring for both patients and caregivers. These groups can be havens of understanding and empathy, where individuals share experiences, discuss challenges, and celebrate milestones together. Let's delve deeper into the avenues to find these groups and the multifaceted benefits they offer.

Discovering the Right Group:
Finding the right support group is akin to discovering a

community that resonates with one's needs and challenges.

- Hospitals and Clinics: Many medical institutions recognize the emotional and psychological challenges associated with kidney disease. They often facilitate support group sessions or can provide references to established local groups.
- National and Local Kidney Organizations: Renowned organizations, like the National Kidney Foundation or the American Association of Kidney Patients, frequently have local chapters or affiliates that conduct support group sessions, workshops, and awareness campaigns.
- Community Centers: Local community hubs, from libraries to religious institutions, often serve as venues for support group meetings. Some even have dedicated boards or sections where such groups advertise their sessions.
- Word of Mouth: Referrals from fellow caregivers, patients, or medical professionals can be invaluable. They offer firsthand insights into the group's dynamics, topics discussed, and overall atmosphere.

Benefits of Joining a Local Support Group:
Beyond just sharing experiences, local support groups provide a spectrum of advantages.

- Educational Opportunities: These groups often invite medical professionals, dietitians, or therapists to impart knowledge about kidney disease management, the latest treatments, or coping strategies.
- Emotional Support: Being surrounded by individuals who truly understand the intricacies of the journey offers emotional solace. It's a space where one can express fears, frustrations, and hopes without judgment.

- Networking: Building relationships with fellow caregivers and patients can lead to discovering new resources, medical recommendations, or even opportunities to participate in relevant events and seminars.
- Shared Resources: From recommending reliable medical professionals to sharing kidney-friendly recipes or local service providers who understand the nuances of the disease, the collective wisdom of the group can be a treasure trove of resources.
- Advocacy and Awareness: As a united front, these groups often participate in awareness campaigns, fundraisers, or events that advocate for kidney disease awareness and patient rights.

Customizing Your Experience:
While the overarching theme of these groups revolves around kidney disease, the experience can be tailored.

- Frequency of Participation: Some may prefer attending meetings regularly, while others might find value in sporadic participation, especially during challenging times.
- Active Participation vs. Observation: While some find solace in actively sharing and discussing, others might benefit merely from listening and being in a supportive environment.
- Specialized Groups: Some local groups might cater specifically to certain demographics, like young adults with kidney disease, pediatric caregivers, or those managing kidney disease alongside other conditions.

Navigating kidney disease's multifaceted challenges becomes more manageable when one is part of a local support group. It provides an anchoring sense of community, a pool of resources, and, most importantly, the reassuring feeling that one is not alone on this journey.

Online Communities

In today's digital age, online communities have emerged as potent platforms offering support, information, and camaraderie to those navigating the challenges of kidney disease. These virtual spaces bridge geographical divides, allowing caregivers and patients from all over the world to connect, share, and uplift each other. However, as with all things on the internet, one must tread with caution, ensuring that the information and advice received are rooted in credible science. Let's delve deeper into how to navigate the vast expanse of online communities effectively.

Social Media Groups:
Platforms like Facebook, Reddit, or LinkedIn are teeming with groups dedicated to kidney disease awareness and support.

- Credibility Check: While many groups provide genuine support, it's essential to exercise caution. Unfortunately, social media is rife with groups pushing fake cures, unproven treatments, or potentially harmful advice. Always cross-check information with credible sources or healthcare professionals.
- Science-backed Groups: Look for groups that emphasize following science and proven medical advice. Groups that regularly feature or reference kidney specialists, doctors, or renal dietitians are usually more reliable.
- Dadvice TV as a Resource: The Dadvice TV YouTube channel and website are excellent examples of credible online resources. And yes, I am biased since I created and run Dadvice TV – but it is all science and fact based. Through interviews with kidney doctors, renal

dietitians, and other kidney specialists, they offer a wealth of knowledge, guidance, and support that aligns with proven science.

Dedicated Forums:
Forums and websites dedicated to kidney health can provide a space for in-depth discussions, advice sharing, and peer support.

- Reputation and Moderation: Opt for forums with a good reputation and active moderation. This ensures that misinformation or potentially harmful advice is kept at bay.
- Patient Testimonies: Reading real-life experiences of those who've walked the kidney disease journey can provide insights, hope, and a sense of community.

Blogs and Podcasts:
Many individuals and organizations document their kidney disease journey or share information via blogs and podcasts.

- Reliability of Information: While personal stories can be insightful, when it comes to medical advice, ensure the blog or podcast cites credible sources or consults with healthcare professionals.
- Guest Features: Blogs or podcasts that feature guest appearances from medical professionals or kidney specialists can be particularly informative. Platforms like Dadvice TV, which regularly interviews experts in the field, serve as trusted resources.

Webinars and Virtual Events:
Many organizations, patient advocacy groups, or health professionals host webinars and virtual events focusing on kidney health.

- Expert Panels: When signing up for webinars, check the list of panelists. Sessions featuring kidney doctors, dietitians, or other medical experts can be particularly

- enlightening.
- Interactive Sessions: Some webinars allow for Q&A sessions, providing an opportunity to get queries addressed by professionals.

Navigating the vast world of online communities can seem daunting. Still, with a discerning eye and a focus on science-backed information, these platforms can offer invaluable support. Whether it's the collective wisdom of a group, the insights from an expert interview on Dadvice TV, or the comfort of reading a fellow patient's blog, the virtual world holds a plethora of resources for those touched by kidney disease.

Family and Friends

The close-knit circle of family and friends often forms the first line of support for those grappling with kidney disease. Their role is multifaceted: they offer emotional solace, practical assistance, and unwavering support during the highs and lows of the journey. Let's explore the depth and breadth of this support system and how to effectively leverage it.

Understanding the Dynamics:
The diagnosis of kidney disease can be overwhelming, not just for the patient but also for their family and friends. Understanding their emotions is the first step toward building a strong support system.

- Educational Sessions: Organizing informal sessions where family and friends can learn about kidney disease can ensure they are well-informed. Knowledge can alleviate fears and misconceptions, enabling them to offer more effective support.
- Empathy and Patience: Recognizing the emotional toll kidney disease can take on the patient and, by extension, the immediate family is crucial. Patience, understanding, and empathy are key in navigating this

journey together.

Seeking Practical Assistance:
The practical challenges of managing kidney disease can be numerous. Fortunately, family and friends can play an instrumental role in mitigating these.

- Shared Responsibilities: Dividing tasks like grocery shopping, cooking kidney-friendly meals, or accompanying the patient to medical appointments can lessen the burden on primary caregivers.
- Creating a Schedule: Using tools like shared calendars can help in organizing tasks, setting reminders for medication, and scheduling doctor visits. This ensures everyone is on the same page.
- Emergency Protocols: Establishing a protocol for emergencies, ensuring a few trusted family members or friends know the necessary steps to take, can provide added reassurance.

Emotional Support and Encouragement:
The emotional and psychological aspects of kidney disease can be as challenging as the physical ones.

- Active Listening: Sometimes, the patient or caregiver just needs someone to listen. Being an active, non-judgmental listener can offer immense emotional relief.
- Recreational Activities: Engaging in light-hearted activities, be it watching a movie, playing a board game, or just reminiscing about fond memories, can offer a temporary respite and boost morale.
- Offering Perspective: In challenging times, a fresh perspective from a trusted family member or friend can make a difference. They can offer hope, positivity, and a reminder of the strength and resilience inherent

in the patient and caregiver.

Regular Check-ins and Updates:
Keeping the wider circle of family and friends updated can ensure continued support and understanding.

- Communication Channels: Establishing regular communication channels, be it through group chats, emails, or periodic gatherings, can keep everyone informed and involved.
- Feedback and Suggestions: Encouraging family and friends to provide feedback or suggestions can lead to discovering new coping strategies, resources, or even medical recommendations.

Family and friends, with their deep-rooted bonds of love and trust, can play an instrumental role in the kidney disease journey. Their unwavering support, both emotional and practical, can be the pillar of strength that both the patient and caregiver lean on during challenging times. By fostering open communication, understanding, and collaboration, this circle can become an invaluable asset in navigating the complexities of kidney disease.

Care for the Caregiver

The role of a caregiver, while immensely rewarding, comes with its unique set of challenges. As they tend to the needs of the kidney patient, it's paramount that caregivers also prioritize their well-being. After all, a caregiver in good health, both physically and mentally, is better equipped to support their loved one effectively. Delving deeper into the manifold aspects of self-care for caregivers, let's explore strategies and approaches to ensure they remain at the pinnacle of their health and well-being.

Understanding the Importance of Self-Care:
Caregivers, in their dedication to their loved ones, often sideline

their own needs. Recognizing the importance of self-care is the foundational step in ensuring their well-being.

- Physical Health: Regular medical check-ups, adhering to a balanced diet, and ensuring adequate rest and sleep are non-negotiable aspects of maintaining good physical health.
- Emotional Well-being: The emotional toll of caregiving can be considerable. Regularly checking in with one's feelings, seeking counseling if needed, and ensuring there are avenues to express emotions are crucial.

Strategies for Effective Self-Care:
Ensuring one's well-being requires a proactive approach. Here are some strategies that can be beneficial:

- Regular Breaks: Intermittently stepping away from caregiving duties, even briefly, can rejuvenate the mind and body. Whether it's a short walk, a hobby, or simply a quiet moment with a book, these breaks can make a significant difference.
- Support Groups for Caregivers: Just as patients benefit from support groups, caregivers too can find solace in groups tailored for their unique challenges. Sharing experiences, seeking advice, or simply being in the company of those who truly understand can be therapeutic.
- Mindfulness and Meditation: Engaging in activities that center the mind, like meditation, yoga, or deep breathing exercises, can help manage stress and offer a sense of tranquility.

Setting Clear Boundaries:
Understanding that one cannot be available 24/7 is vital for a caregiver's mental and emotional health.

- Delegating Tasks: Caregivers needn't shoulder all

responsibilities alone. Enlisting the help of other family members or even hiring professional help for specific tasks can distribute the load.
- Communicating Needs: Being vocal about one's limits, needs, and seeking assistance when required can ensure that the caregiver doesn't get overwhelmed.

Engaging in Recreational Activities:
Activities unrelated to caregiving can offer a refreshing change of pace and perspective.

- Pursuing Hobbies: Be it painting, music, gardening, or any other hobby, setting aside time for activities that bring joy can be incredibly therapeutic.
- Social Connections: Maintaining social ties, catching up with friends, or participating in group activities can provide a much-needed emotional boost.

Seeking Professional Guidance:
At times, the challenges of caregiving might necessitate professional intervention.

- Counseling and Therapy: Regular sessions with a counselor or therapist can provide coping strategies, emotional support, and an avenue to discuss challenges without judgment.
- Educational Workshops: Attending workshops or seminars designed for caregivers can provide new perspectives, strategies, and tools to manage the multifaceted challenges of caregiving.

Being a beacon of support for someone with kidney disease is a role of paramount importance. But as the adage goes, "You cannot pour from an empty cup." Caregivers must ensure their cup remains full, not just for the sake of the ones they care for but for their own well-being and fulfillment. With the right strategies, support, and self-awareness, caregivers can ensure they remain at their best, ready to face the challenges and joys of the caregiving journey.

THE PATH FORWARD

The journey through kidney disease is one of constant learning, adaptation, and evolution. For caregivers, it is a path intertwined with emotions ranging from fear to hope, from despair to determination. But amidst the unpredictability and challenges, there remains a steadfast beacon of hope: the indomitable human spirit. This chapter seeks to offer a guiding light, focusing on the inherent resilience of families, the actionable steps to enhance the caregiving journey, and the profound impact a caregiver can have on their loved one's life.

The Resilience Factor

Resilience, often termed as the backbone of human spirit, embodies the capability to weather the storms of life and emerge not only unbroken but often stronger. In the context of kidney disease, it's this very resilience, especially within a family unit, that can turn the tide. But what does resilience look like in action?

- Shared Strength: Every family has a unique dynamic, a special bond that holds them together. Drawing strength from one another during tough times becomes paramount. Reflecting on my journey, I remember being told I wouldn't live more than 45 days without Dialysis. It was the unwavering support of my family, their belief in my strength, and our collective determination that empowered me to leverage diet and lifestyle changes, effectively staving off the need for

dialysis for years.
- Adaptive Coping Mechanisms: Families learn to evolve and adapt. When I was first diagnosed, my children, despite their young age, were incredibly active in helping me spread the importance of early detection of kidney disease. Their involvement not only helped raise awareness but also gave our family a collective purpose, a mission to work towards.
- Empowerment through Knowledge: The thirst for knowledge can be a driving force. I personally delved deep into understanding kidney disease, which led to the creation of Dadvice TV, a platform where kidney experts, renal dietitians, and personal experiences come together. This became not just a source of empowerment for me but also a beacon of hope for many.
- Celebrating Milestones: Every achievement, no matter how small, deserves to be celebrated. Whether it was learning to enjoy a plant-based meal without craving a ribeye steak or being able to walk to the mailbox and back without getting out of breath, each milestone brought renewed hope and was a testament to our resilience.

In the battle against kidney disease, resilience emerges as both shield and spear. It's not just about enduring; it's about thriving, evolving, and making a difference. Through personal endeavors, shared efforts, and an undying spirit, families can indeed turn challenges into opportunities, crafting a narrative of hope and triumph.

Next Steps

Equipping oneself with the right set of tools and resources is like arming oneself for a journey. It's about preparation, foresight, and having a proactive mindset. With kidney disease, every informed action taken can be a step towards better health and improved quality of life. Here's a deeper dive into the actionable steps caregivers can consider.

- Stay Updated: Medicine and healthcare are rapidly evolving fields. Today's research could become tomorrow's groundbreaking treatment. Subscribing to medical journals, attending conferences, or simply setting up Google alerts for kidney health news can ensure you're in the loop. For instance, new research might shed light on beneficial dietary components or innovative treatment modalities.
- Utilize Technology: The digital era offers a plethora of tools tailored to assist caregivers. Apps that remind of medication schedules, telehealth platforms that allow consultations from the comfort of home, and even online platforms like Dadvice TV, which brings expert opinions and advice to your fingertips, are invaluable resources.
- Engage with the Medical Team: Open channels of communication with the medical team are crucial. Regularly scheduled check-ins, be it for routine tests or discussions about the patient's progress, can provide clarity and direction. Don't hesitate to ask questions; understanding the nuances of the condition can empower caregivers to make more informed decisions.
- Access Support Systems: The support system for kidney disease is vast and varied. From dedicated kidney foundations to online forums, there's a wealth of resources out there. Local workshops, often organized by healthcare institutions or patient advocacy groups, can provide hands-on training or guidance on specific caregiving challenges.
- Educational Endeavors: Knowledge truly is power.

Consider enrolling in courses or workshops that delve deeper into kidney health, dietary needs, or even psychological care. Institutions often offer courses tailored for caregivers, focusing on both the medical and emotional aspects of care.
- Plan for the Future: As with any long-term condition, planning ahead is essential. This includes discussions about potential treatment paths, understanding the progression of the disease, and even discussing the financial aspects, from insurance to potential costs of treatments.
- Seek Holistic Approaches: While medical care is paramount, holistic approaches can complement it. Research on the benefits of therapies like massage, acupuncture, or even meditation, and see if they can be integrated into the care regimen. Always consult with the medical team before introducing any new element to ensure it's safe and beneficial.

The journey of caregiving in the context of kidney disease is undoubtedly complex. But with the right steps, resources, and a proactive approach, it's a journey that can be navigated with confidence and hope. Each action taken, every piece of knowledge acquired, adds a layer of strength, ensuring that caregivers are well-prepared to face challenges and celebrate milestones.

Your Role

How You Make a Difference:
Being a caregiver is not just a title or a role; it's a beacon of hope, a shoulder to lean on, and often the very lifeline that anchors a kidney patient to the shores of optimism. If you're reading this, you've taken on an immensely significant responsibility, and for that, heartfelt gratitude is in order.
- **A Heartfelt Thank You**: First and foremost, a

resounding thank you for stepping into this role. It's not a path many choose, and your decision to be a guiding light speaks volumes about your compassion, strength, and commitment. Kidney patients, like many with chronic conditions, often find themselves on a journey that doesn't garner the limelight, making your involvement even more crucial.

- Being the Anchor: Kidney disease, despite its prevalence, doesn't always receive the attention or awareness it warrants. Patients can often feel overshadowed, lost in the vastness of the medical world. Your presence, your willingness to understand, learn, and support can change this narrative. Your role can shift a patient's perspective from feeling isolated to feeling cherished and understood.
- Beyond Medical Support: While managing appointments, medications, and diets are tangible aspects of caregiving, the intangibles often make the most significant difference. Simple acts like listening, offering words of encouragement, or just being there can transform a patient's day. Remember, it's not always about 'doing'; sometimes, it's about 'being'.
- Championing Their Cause: Advocacy goes beyond attending medical appointments. It's about raising awareness, fighting for their rights, and ensuring they get the care and attention they deserve. Your voice can amplify their concerns, making sure they don't get lost in the din.
- The Power of Positivity: Having a caregiver to share the journey can be the difference between merely existing and truly thriving. Your optimism, your belief in better days, can infuse hope, making the challenging days more manageable and the good days even more joyful.

Your role as a caregiver, dear reader, is akin to a lighthouse, guiding kidney patients through turbulent waters towards safer shores. The magnitude of your contribution cannot be encapsulated in mere words. Through your actions, commitment, and sheer presence, you're offering one of the greatest gifts – the gift of hope and unwavering support. As you walk this path, know that each step you take is creating ripples of positive change, making the kidney disease journey one of resilience, hope, and collective strength.

Farewell Note

As this chapter draws to a close, it's essential to pause, reflect, and truly appreciate the journey you've embarked upon. Your decision to be a caregiver, to be that beacon of hope in a kidney patient's life, is a testament to the immense strength, compassion, and love within you.

Your commitment to understanding and supporting a loved one with kidney disease will undoubtedly bring forth challenges, but intertwined with these challenges will be moments of profound connection, joy, and growth. The path ahead will be one of learning – not just about the intricacies of kidney disease, but also about the depths of human resilience, the power of community, and the boundless capacity of the human heart to care, nurture, and uplift.

As you forge ahead, remember that you are not alone on this journey. The subsequent sections of this book are filled with a plethora of resources, meticulously curated to assist you every step of the way. From comprehensive insights into various facets of kidney disease to a glossary of terms designed to enhance your understanding, the information ahead aims to empower you with knowledge and confidence.

Navigating kidney disease, while undeniably complex, is a journey that can be filled with hope and positivity, especially with dedicated caregivers like you leading the way. As you turn the pages ahead, may you continue to find insights, inspiration, and the unwavering belief that together, we can conquer the challenges and embrace the joys that life has to offer.

Remember, each day is a new chapter, filled with opportunities, learning, and love. Here's to writing a story that resonates with hope, strength, and the undying human spirit. Farewell for now, dear reader, and onward to the journey ahead. You got this!

UNDERSTANDING LABS AND DIAGNOSTICS

Regular monitoring of kidney function and associated markers is essential for individuals with chronic kidney disease (CKD). Proper interpretation of laboratory tests and diagnostic tools can help identify the progression of the disease, evaluate the effectiveness of treatments, and detect potential complications. This chapter will discuss the key laboratory tests and diagnostic tools used in the assessment and management of CKD, as well as the importance of understanding these results for optimal disease management.

Blood Tests

Several blood tests are used to monitor kidney function, detect potential complications, and assess overall health in individuals with CKD. These tests include:

1. Estimated glomerular filtration rate (eGFR): The eGFR is a measure of kidney function and is calculated using a blood test for creatinine, a waste product that is removed from the blood by the kidneys. The eGFR is expressed in milliliters per minute per 1.73 square meters (mL/min/1.73 m^2) and is adjusted for age, sex, and race. An eGFR below 60 for three months or more indicates CKD. The eGFR is used to classify CKD into five stages, with

lower values indicating more advanced disease.

2. Blood urea nitrogen (BUN): BUN is another waste product that is removed from the blood by the kidneys. Elevated BUN levels may indicate reduced kidney function, dehydration, or other factors that can affect kidney function.

3. Complete blood count (CBC): The CBC provides information about the number and types of cells in the blood, including red blood cells, white blood cells, and platelets. This test is used to assess overall health, detect anemia (a common complication of CKD), and monitor the response to treatments for anemia.

4. Electrolytes: The kidneys play a crucial role in maintaining the balance of electrolytes in the body, such as sodium, potassium, calcium, and phosphorus. Blood tests for electrolytes can help identify imbalances that may be indicative of CKD or potential complications, such as hyperkalemia (high potassium levels) or hyperphosphatemia (high phosphorus levels).

5. Parathyroid hormone (PTH): PTH is a hormone that helps regulate calcium and phosphorus levels in the body. Elevated PTH levels can be a sign of bone and mineral disorders in individuals with CKD, as the kidneys may struggle to maintain the balance of these minerals.

6. Albumin: Albumin is a protein found in the blood that helps maintain fluid balance and transport substances throughout the body. Low albumin levels may be a sign of malnutrition or inflammation in individuals with CKD.

Urine Tests

Urine tests are used to assess kidney function, detect potential complications, and evaluate the effectiveness of treatments for CKD. These tests include:

1. Urinalysis: A urinalysis involves a physical, chemical, and microscopic examination of a urine sample. This test can help detect abnormalities in the urine, such as the presence of blood (hematuria), excess protein (proteinuria), or signs of infection.

2. Urine albumin-to-creatinine ratio (UACR): The UACR is a measure of the amount of albumin (a protein) in the urine, which can be an early indicator of kidney damage. A UACR of 30 mg/g or higher is considered abnormal and may indicate CKD.

3. 24-hour urine collection: A 24-hour urine collection involves collecting all urine produced over a 24-hour period to measure the total volume of urine and assess the levels of various substances, such as protein or creatinine. This test can provide more accurate information about kidney function and help detect potential complications in individuals with CKD.

Imaging Studies

Imaging studies can be used to evaluate the size, shape, and structure of the kidneys, detect potential complications, or identify the underlying cause of CKD. These studies include:

1. Ultrasound: An ultrasound is a non-invasive imaging technique that uses sound waves to create images of the kidneys. This test can help detect structural abnormalities, such as kidney stones, cysts, or tumors, as well as assess blood flow to the kidneys.

2. Computed tomography (CT) scan: A CT scan is an imaging technique that uses X-rays and a computer to create detailed, cross-sectional images of the kidneys. This test can help detect structural abnormalities, such as kidney stones, cysts, or tumors, as well as assess blood flow to the kidneys. A CT scan may be performed with or without contrast, depending on the clinical situation and the individual's risk factors.

3. Magnetic resonance imaging (MRI): An MRI is an imaging technique that uses a magnetic field and radio waves to create detailed, cross-sectional images of the kidneys. This test can help detect structural abnormalities, such as kidney stones, cysts, or tumors, as well as assess blood flow to the kidneys. An MRI may be performed with or without contrast, depending on the clinical situation and the individual's risk factors.

Kidney Biopsy

A kidney biopsy is a medical procedure that involves obtaining a small sample of kidney tissue for examination under a microscope. This is typically done to diagnose kidney disease, determine the severity of the condition, or evaluate how well a treatment plan is working. During a kidney biopsy, a needle is inserted through the skin and into the kidney to collect the tissue sample. The procedure is usually performed under local anesthesia and may involve the use of ultrasound or other imaging techniques to help guide the needle to the appropriate location. The collected tissue is then analyzed by a pathologist to provide valuable information about the health and function of the kidneys.

IMPORTANT LAB TEST VALUES

As a kidney patient caregiver, it is helpful to familiarize yourself with the essential lab tests that monitor kidney function and overall health. By understanding these tests and their normal ranges, you will be better equipped to track your loved ones progress, communicate with their healthcare team, and make informed decisions about their treatment plan. In this chapter, we will cover some of the most important lab tests for kidney patients, discuss their normal ranges, and explain what each test measures.

Albumin

Normal Range: 3.4-5.4 g/dL

Albumin is a protein made by the liver that helps maintain fluid balance and transports various substances through the bloodstream. Low albumin levels can indicate malnutrition or inflammation, both of which are common in kidney disease. Ensuring proper protein intake and managing inflammation can help maintain healthy albumin levels.

Blood Urea Nitrogen (BUN)

Normal Range: 7-20 mg/dL

BUN measures the amount of nitrogen in your blood that comes from the waste product urea, which is created when your body breaks down proteins. High BUN levels can indicate reduced kidney function, as the kidneys are less able to remove urea from the bloodstream. Treatment may involve adjusting protein intake, managing other health conditions, or altering medications.

Calcium

Normal Range: 8.6-10.2 mg/dL

Calcium is essential for strong bones, blood clotting, and proper nerve and muscle function. Kidney patients often experience imbalances in calcium levels, which can lead to bone disease, heart problems, or other complications. Treatment may involve dietary changes, medications, or dialysis adjustments.

Creatinine

Normal Range: Males - 0.74-1.35 mg/dL; Females - 0.59-1.04 mg/dL

Creatinine is a waste product that comes from the normal wear and tear on muscles in the body. High creatinine levels can indicate reduced kidney function, as the kidneys are less able to filter creatinine from the blood. Treatment may involve managing underlying health conditions, medications, or adjusting dialysis if applicable.

Estimated Glomerular Filtration Rate (eGFR)

Normal Range: >90 mL/min/1.73 m²

eGFR is a calculation based on your creatinine level, age, sex, and race that estimates how well your kidneys are filtering waste from your blood. Lower eGFR values can indicate worsening kidney function, and treatment may involve managing underlying health conditions, medications, or dialysis if necessary. Your eGFR is NOT a static number and can fluctuate throughout the day, so focus on the trend and not a single value. It is natural for your eGFR to decline by approximately 1 point each year after 40.

Hematocrit (HCT)

Normal Range: Males - 38.8-50%; Females - 34.9-44.5%

Hematocrit measures the proportion of red blood cells in

your blood. A low HCT can indicate anemia, a common complication in kidney disease, as the kidneys produce less of the hormone erythropoietin, which stimulates red blood cell production. Treating anemia may involve iron supplementation, erythropoiesis-stimulating agents, or blood transfusions.

Hemoglobin

Normal Range: Males - 13.5-17.5 g/dL; Females: 12.0-15.5 g/dL

Hemoglobin is an essential component of red blood cells that carries oxygen from your lungs to the rest of your body. Low hemoglobin levels (anemia) are common in kidney disease, as the kidneys produce a hormone called erythropoietin, which stimulates red blood cell production. Anemia can cause fatigue, weakness, and shortness of breath.

A1c (A1c)

Normal Range: 4-5.6%

The A1c test measures your average blood sugar levels over the past 2-3 months. High A1c levels can indicate poor blood sugar control in people with diabetes, a major risk factor for kidney disease. Maintaining proper blood sugar control is essential for preventing or managing kidney damage in diabetic patients.

High-Density Lipoprotein (HDL)

Normal Range: Males - >40 mg/dL; Females - >50 mg/dL

HDL cholesterol is often called "good" cholesterol because it helps remove harmful cholesterol from the bloodstream, reducing the risk of heart disease. Higher levels of HDL are generally considered better for heart health.

Low-Density Lipoprotein (LDL)

Normal Range: <100 mg/dL

LDL cholesterol is often called "bad" cholesterol because it contributes to the buildup of plaque in the arteries, increasing the risk of heart disease. Lowering LDL levels can be achieved through lifestyle changes and medications, if necessary.

Phosphorus

Normal Range: 2.5-4.5 mg/dL

Phosphorus is a mineral that works with calcium to help build strong bones and teeth. In kidney disease, the kidneys may have difficulty removing excess phosphorus from the blood, leading to high levels that can cause bone and heart problems. Managing phosphorus levels may involve dietary changes, phosphate binders, or adjustments to dialysis.

Potassium

Normal Range: 3.5-5.0 mEq/L

Potassium is an essential mineral that helps maintain proper nerve and muscle function, including the heart. In kidney disease, the kidneys may struggle to maintain normal potassium levels, leading to imbalances that can cause irregular heartbeats or other complications. Treatment may involve dietary changes, medications, or dialysis adjustments.

Red Blood Cells (RBC)

Normal Range: Males - 4.7-6.1 million cells/mcL; Females - 4.2-5.4 million cells/mcL

Red blood cells carry oxygen from the lungs to the rest of the body and remove carbon dioxide. A low RBC count can indicate anemia, a common complication in kidney disease. Treatment for anemia may involve iron supplementation, erythropoiesis-stimulating agents, or blood transfusions.

Sodium

Normal Range: 135-145 mEq/L

Sodium is an essential electrolyte that helps maintain fluid balance and proper nerve and muscle function. Imbalances in sodium levels can occur in kidney disease, leading to complications such as high blood pressure or fluid retention. Treatment may involve dietary changes, medications, or dialysis adjustments.

Total Cholesterol (TC)

Normal Range: <200 mg/dL

Total cholesterol is a measure of the cholesterol in your blood, including both "good" (HDL) and "bad" (LDL) cholesterol. High total cholesterol levels can increase the risk of heart disease, and managing cholesterol levels is important for overall cardiovascular health.

Triglycerides

Normal Range: <150 mg/dL

Triglycerides are a type of fat found in your blood that your body uses for energy. High triglyceride levels can increase the risk of heart disease. Lowering triglycerides may involve lifestyle changes, such as diet and exercise, or medications if necessary.

Uric Acid

Normal Range: Males - 3.4-7.0 mg/dL; Females - 2.4-6.0 mg/dL

Uric acid is a waste product that results from the breakdown of purines, which are found in certain foods and produced by the body. High uric acid levels can lead to gout or kidney stones and may be associated with reduced kidney function. Treatment may involve dietary changes, medications, or managing underlying health conditions.

Vitamin D

Normal Range: 20-50 ng/mL

Vitamin D is essential for maintaining strong bones and a healthy immune system. In kidney disease, the kidneys may struggle to activate vitamin D, leading to low levels that can contribute to bone disease or other complications. Treatment may involve vitamin D supplementation, managing phosphorus and calcium levels, or adjusting dialysis if applicable.

Understanding and keeping track of these lab tests and their values is crucial for kidney patients. By staying informed about lab test results, you can work closely with the healthcare team to make the best decisions regarding your loved ones treatment plan and lifestyle adjustments. Remember, knowledge is power, and being proactive in managing kidney health can significantly improve your loved ones quality of life and outcomes.

GLOSSARY OF TERMS AND DEFINITIONS

Here's an extensive glossary of kidney-related terms and definitions to help readers familiarize themselves with the language of CKD:

Acidosis: A condition characterized by an excess of acid in the blood, which can cause a variety of symptoms and complications. Acidosis is common in people with kidney disease because the kidneys are responsible for maintaining the body's acid-base balance.

Acute Kidney Injury (AKI): A sudden and temporary loss of kidney function, which can be caused by various factors, such as severe infection, trauma, or medication side effects. AKI can be reversible if treated promptly, but may also lead to chronic kidney disease (CKD) or kidney failure.

Anemia: A condition characterized by a decrease in the number of red blood cells or a decrease in the amount of hemoglobin in the blood. Anemia can cause fatigue, shortness of breath, and other symptoms. It is common in people with kidney disease due to reduced production of the hormone erythropoietin, which stimulates red blood cell production.

Arteriovenous (AV) Fistula: A type of vascular access for hemodialysis that involves connecting an artery directly to a vein, typically in the arm. This creates a high-flow connection that can withstand the pressure of the dialysis machine and provides long-lasting access to the bloodstream.

Automated Peritoneal Dialysis (APD): A form of peritoneal dialysis that uses a machine to automatically exchange the dialysis fluid in the patient's abdominal cavity, typically overnight while the patient sleeps.

Azotemia: A condition characterized by high levels of nitrogen-containing waste products in the blood, such as urea and creatinine. Azotemia can occur in people with reduced kidney function or kidney failure.

Bicarbonate: A substance that helps to neutralize acid in the blood and maintain the body's acid-base balance. People with kidney disease may have low bicarbonate levels, leading to acidosis.

Catheter: A type of vascular access for hemodialysis that involves inserting a long, thin tube (catheter) into a large vein, usually in the neck or chest. Catheters are generally used as a temporary access option when a fistula or graft is not available or is not functioning properly. They have a higher risk of infection and other complications compared to fistulas and grafts.

Chronic Kidney Disease (CKD): A long-term condition characterized by the gradual loss of kidney function over time, which can lead to kidney failure if not treated. CKD can be caused by a variety of factors, such as diabetes, hypertension, and autoimmune diseases.

Continuous Ambulatory Peritoneal Dialysis (CAPD): A form of peritoneal dialysis in which the patient manually exchanges the dialysis fluid in their abdominal cavity several times per day, without the need for a machine.

Creatinine: A waste product that is produced by the normal breakdown of muscle tissue and is removed from the body by the kidneys. Elevated creatinine levels in the blood can be a sign of reduced kidney function.

Dehydration: A condition in which the body does not have

enough water to maintain proper fluid balance and support overall health. Dehydration can cause a variety of symptoms and complications, including kidney damage, and is particularly dangerous for people with kidney disease.

Diabetes: A chronic disease characterized by high blood sugar levels due to the body's inability to produce or effectively use insulin. Diabetes is the leading cause of chronic kidney disease and kidney failure.

Dialysis: A medical treatment that uses a machine to remove waste products and excess fluid from the blood when the kidneys are no longer able to function properly. There are two main types of dialysis: hemodialysis and peritoneal dialysis.

Dialysis Adequacy: A measure of how effectively dialysis is removing waste products and excess fluid from the blood. Adequacy is assessed through regular blood tests and is an important factor in determining the frequency and duration of dialysis treatments.

Diuretics: Medications that help the body get rid of excess fluid by increasing urine production. Diuretics are often used to treat high blood pressure and fluid retention in people with kidney disease.

Donor: A person who provides an organ, such as a kidney, for transplantation. Donors can be living (usually a close relative or friend) or deceased (someone who has died and agreed to donate their organs).

Edema: Swelling caused by excess fluid trapped in the body's tissues, often affecting the legs, ankles, and feet. Edema is a common symptom of kidney disease and can be managed through medications, dietary changes, and other treatments.

Electrolytes: Minerals in the body, such as sodium, potassium, and calcium, that have an electric charge and play crucial roles in maintaining the body's fluid balance, nerve function, and muscle function. Electrolyte imbalances are common in people with kidney disease and can cause a variety of symptoms and complications.

Erythropoiesis-Stimulating Agents (ESAs): Synthetic forms of erythropoietin used to treat anemia in people with kidney disease. These medications stimulate red blood cell production and can help improve symptoms of anemia.

Erythropoietin (EPO): A hormone produced by the kidneys that stimulates the production of red blood cells. People with kidney disease may have reduced EPO production, leading to anemia.

Fistula: A type of vascular access for hemodialysis that involves connecting an artery directly to a vein, typically in the arm. This creates a high-flow connection that can withstand the pressure of the dialysis machine and provides long-lasting access to the bloodstream.

GFR (Glomerular Filtration Rate): A measure of how well the kidneys are filtering waste and excess fluid from the blood. A lower GFR indicates reduced kidney function, with a GFR below 60 considered chronic kidney disease and a GFR below 15 considered kidney failure.

Graft: A type of vascular access for hemodialysis that involves connecting an artery to a vein using a synthetic tube, typically when a fistula is not possible or has failed. Grafts are more prone to infection and clotting than fistulas, but they can provide a reliable access option for some patients.

Hematuria: The presence of blood in the urine, which can be a sign of kidney disease or other medical conditions. Hematuria can be visible to the naked eye (gross hematuria) or only detectable under a microscope (microscopic hematuria).

Hemodialysis: A type of dialysis that uses a machine to filter waste products and excess fluid from the blood through an artificial kidney (dialyzer). Hemodialysis is typically performed in a dialysis center or hospital, usually three times per week.

Hypercalcemia: A condition characterized by high levels of

calcium in the blood. Hypercalcemia can cause a variety of symptoms and complications, including kidney stones and bone disease. It is common in people with advanced kidney disease due to impaired calcium regulation by the kidneys.

Hyperkalemia: A condition characterized by high levels of potassium in the blood. Hyperkalemia can cause muscle weakness, irregular heartbeat, and other symptoms, and can be life-threatening if not treated promptly. It is a common complication of kidney disease and can be managed through diet and medication.

Hyperphosphatemia: A condition characterized by high levels of phosphate in the blood. Hyperphosphatemia is common in people with kidney disease because the kidneys are responsible for filtering excess phosphate from the blood. It can contribute to bone disease and cardiovascular problems.

Hypertension: A condition characterized by consistently high blood pressure, which can damage blood vessels and organs, including the kidneys. Hypertension is both a cause and a complication of kidney disease and requires careful management through lifestyle changes and medications.

Hypocalcemia: A condition characterized by low levels of calcium in the blood. Hypocalcemia can cause muscle cramps, numbness, and other symptoms. It can be a result of certain medications or dietary imbalances and can be managed through diet and supplementation.

Hypokalemia: A condition characterized by low levels of potassium in the blood. Hypokalemia can cause muscle weakness, fatigue, and irregular heartbeat. It can be a result of certain medications or dietary imbalances and can be managed through diet and supplementation.

Hypophosphatemia: A condition characterized by low levels of phosphate in the blood. Hypophosphatemia can cause muscle weakness, bone pain, and other symptoms. It can be a result of certain medications or dietary imbalances and can be managed through diet and supplementation.

IgA Nephropathy: A kidney disease caused by the buildup of the antibody immunoglobulin A (IgA) in the kidneys, leading to inflammation and reduced kidney function. IgA nephropathy is one of the most common causes of glomerulonephritis, and treatment may include medications to manage blood pressure and reduce inflammation.

Kidney Biopsy: A medical procedure in which a small sample of kidney tissue is removed, usually with a needle, for examination under a microscope. A kidney biopsy can help diagnose the cause of kidney disease and guide treatment decisions.

Kidney Failure: The final stage of chronic kidney disease, in which the kidneys are no longer able to filter waste products and excess fluid from the blood. Kidney failure requires treatment with dialysis or a kidney transplant to sustain life.

Kidney Stone: A hard, crystalline mass that forms in the kidneys from substances in the urine, such as calcium, oxalate, and phosphate. Kidney stones can cause severe pain and other symptoms and may require treatment with medications, dietary changes, or surgical intervention.

Kidney Transplant: A surgical procedure in which a healthy kidney from a donor is implanted into a person with kidney failure. A kidney transplant can provide improved quality of life and longer survival compared to dialysis, but it requires lifelong immunosuppressive medications to prevent rejection.

Lupus Nephritis: Kidney inflammation caused by the autoimmune disease lupus, which can lead to kidney damage and reduced kidney function. Treatment for lupus nephritis involves managing the underlying lupus and may include medications to suppress the immune system.

Nephrectomy: The surgical removal of a kidney, usually due to severe damage or cancer. In some cases, a person can live with one functioning kidney, while in others, dialysis or a kidney transplant may be necessary.

Nephritic Syndrome: A group of symptoms and signs caused by inflammation of the glomeruli in the kidneys, leading to reduced kidney function. Nephritic syndrome can include hematuria, hypertension, and reduced urine output.

Nephrologist: A medical specialist who focuses on diagnosing and treating diseases and disorders of the kidneys.

Nephrotic Syndrome: A kidney disorder characterized by high levels of protein in the urine, low levels of protein in the blood, and swelling (edema) due to fluid retention. Nephrotic syndrome can be caused by a variety of underlying conditions, such as diabetes or autoimmune diseases, and can lead to progressive kidney damage if not treated.

Peritoneal Dialysis (PD): A type of dialysis that uses the patient's own peritoneal membrane (lining of the abdominal cavity) as a filter to remove waste products and excess fluid from the blood. PD is typically performed at home, with the patient manually or automatically exchanging dialysis fluid in their abdominal cavity.

Polycystic Kidney Disease (PKD): A genetic disorder that causes numerous fluid-filled cysts to form in the kidneys, leading to enlarged kidneys and reduced kidney function. PKD is the most common inherited cause of kidney disease and can eventually lead to kidney failure.

Potassium: An electrolyte that plays a crucial role in maintaining the body's fluid balance, nerve function, and muscle function. Potassium levels must be carefully managed in people with kidney disease, as both high and low levels can cause serious complications.

Proteinuria: The presence of excess protein in the urine, which can be a sign of kidney disease or other medical conditions. Proteinuria can cause foamy urine and may require treatment with medications or dietary changes.

Renal: Pertaining to the kidneys.

Renal Diet: A specialized diet designed for people with kidney disease, which typically involves controlling the intake of sodium, potassium, phosphorus, and protein to help manage symptoms and slow the progression of kidney disease.

Renal Osteodystrophy: A bone disorder that occurs in people with chronic kidney disease, caused by imbalances in calcium, phosphorus, and parathyroid hormone. Renal osteodystrophy can lead to weak, brittle bones and may require treatment with medications and dietary changes.

Sodium: An electrolyte that plays a crucial role in maintaining the body's fluid balance, nerve function, and muscle function. Sodium levels must be carefully managed in people with kidney disease, as both high and low levels can cause serious complications.

Transplant: A surgical procedure in which a healthy organ from a donor is implanted into a person with organ failure. A kidney transplant is a treatment option for people with kidney failure that can provide improved quality of life and longer survival compared to dialysis.

Urea: A waste product that is produced by the breakdown of proteins in the body and is removed by the kidneys. Elevated levels of urea in the blood can be a sign of reduced kidney function.

Uremia: A condition characterized by high levels of waste products in the blood, such as urea and creatinine, due to reduced kidney function or kidney failure. Uremia can cause a variety of symptoms and complications, including fatigue, nausea, and shortness of breath.

Urinalysis: A laboratory test that examines the chemical and microscopic properties of a urine sample to help diagnose kidney disease and other medical conditions.

Urinary Tract Infection (UTI): An infection in any part of the urinary system, including the kidneys, bladder, or urethra. UTIs are more common in people with kidney disease and can cause pain, fever, and other symptoms.

Urine Output: The amount of urine produced by the kidneys, which can be used to assess kidney function and hydration status. Reduced urine output can be a sign of kidney disease, dehydration, or other medical conditions.

Vascular Access: A method of connecting a patient's bloodstream to a dialysis machine, allowing for the removal of waste products and excess fluid. Common types of vascular access for hemodialysis include arteriovenous fistulas, grafts, and catheters.

Vascular Calcification: and can contribute to cardiovascular complications, such as high blood pressure, heart disease, and stroke. Management of vascular calcification in kidney disease may involve medications, dietary changes, and addressing other risk factors, such as high blood pressure and diabetes.

Vasculitis: Inflammation of the blood vessels, which can cause them to narrow, weaken, or leak. Vasculitis can affect the kidneys and other organs, leading to reduced kidney function or kidney failure. Treatment for vasculitis may include medications to reduce inflammation and suppress the immune system.

Vitamin D: A fat-soluble vitamin that plays a crucial role in maintaining healthy bones, immune function, and overall health. People with kidney disease often have low levels of vitamin D due to impaired kidney function and may require supplementation or treatment with activated vitamin D to maintain normal levels.

Water Intake: The amount of water consumed by a person, which can affect kidney function and overall health. People with kidney disease may need to carefully manage their water intake to prevent dehydration or fluid overload, depending on their individual needs and stage of kidney disease.

Water Retention: The accumulation of excess fluid in the body, often causing swelling (edema) in the legs, ankles, and feet. Water retention is a common symptom of kidney disease and can be managed through medications, dietary changes, and other treatments.

ABOUT THE AUTHOR

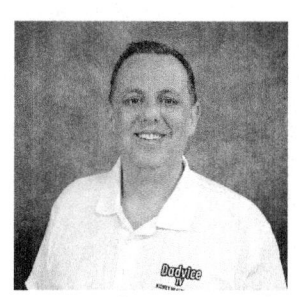

James Fabin

James Fabin is a devoted husband and loving father of two young children. Throughout his life, James has been an active participant in charitable endeavors, dedicating his time and resources to make a positive impact on the lives of others.

A passionate animal lover, James shares his home with two beloved dogs and volunteers with animal rescue groups, providing support and assistance to animals in need. His dedication to helping others, whether they have two legs or four, is evident in everything he does.

In his professional life, James works in the automotive industry, where he specializes in marketing. His expertise in this field has allowed him to connect with people from all walks of life and apply his skills to create meaningful and lasting relationships.

James's journey with chronic kidney disease has inspired him to share his knowledge and experience with others, providing valuable insights and practical advice through his writing. By combining his passion for helping others with his personal experiences, James hopes to empower those facing kidney disease to take control of their health and improve their quality of life.

Learn more about James and watch his ever-growing kidney video library at www.DadviceTV.com

BOOKS BY THIS AUTHOR

Conquering Kidney Disease: A Survivors Guide To Thriving With Ckd

Embark on a comprehensive journey through the world of kidney health with this definitive guide that intertwines scientific insight, practical advice, and a compassionate approach to managing kidney disease. This book is an invaluable resource for anyone who's grappling with the challenges of kidney disease, kidney failure, or simply wishes to understand the intricacies of kidney health better.

Discover the answers to your pressing questions about kidney disease, from its earliest stages to the potential of kidney failure. Learn the importance of early detection, understand how the disease progresses, and uncover the power of proactive management of your health. With detailed explanations made easy to understand, you'll gain a solid grasp of what chronic kidney disease (CKD) entails.

The book goes beyond just medical facts and delves into the everyday realities of living with kidney disease, offering practical advice on maintaining a kidney-friendly lifestyle. Central to this is the kidney diet. This book dispels the one-size-fits-all myth, emphasizing that a kidney diet should be as unique as you are. You'll learn about the significance of protein in your diet, the differences between animal and plant proteins, and how the right balance can help manage your condition.

Master the art of individualized diet planning with help from experts and real-life stories. This book encourages a collaborative care approach, urging the involvement of renal dietitians and healthcare teams in managing your kidney health. Explore different treatment options, including dialysis and kidney transplants, helping you make informed decisions about your health journey.

Armed with the latest research, personal anecdotes, and a wealth of practical tips, this book aims to inspire, educate, and empower you to take control of your kidney health. Whether you are a kidney patient yourself, a caretaker, or a health professional seeking to enhance your knowledge, this comprehensive guide presents a holistic view of kidney health. Navigate the landscape of kidney disease with confidence, armed with knowledge, and inspired to make the best choices for your unique journey.

Conquering The Kidney Diet: Thriving With Ckd Through Nutrition

Embark on a transformative journey towards thriving with CKD through the power of nutrition. In "Conquering the Kidney Diet," the highly anticipated second book by James Fabin, you will find the keys to unlocking the potential of the kidney diet and embracing a life of vitality. This empowering guide is specifically designed for individuals not currently on dialysis, providing you with essential knowledge and practical advice to navigate the kidney diet with confidence and clarity. Say goodbye to fear and uncertainty as you discover how to dine out, enjoy social gatherings, and make informed choices that support your kidney health. Unlike conventional approaches that limit your options, this book transforms the way you approach your kidney diet.

Printed in Great Britain
by Amazon